NO
HARM
DONE

THREE PLAYS ABOUT
MEDICAL CONDITIONS

NO HARM DONE

THREE PLAYS ABOUT MEDICAL CONDITIONS

—᚜᚜—

EUGENE STICKLAND

DURVILE &
UpRoute Books

Calgary, Alberta, Canada

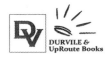

Durvile & UpRoute Books

UPROUTE IMPRINT OF DURVILE PUBLICATIONS LTD.

Calgary, Alberta, Canada
Durvile.com

LIBRARY AND ARCHIVES CATALOGUING IN PUBLICATIONS DATA

No Harm Done: Three Plays about Medical Conditions
Stickland, Eugene, author

1. Health Care Issues
2. Theatre | 3. Performing Arts | 4. Playwriting

Every River Lit Series. Series editor, Lorene Shyba

978-1-988824-70-3 (pbk)
978-1-988824-71-0 (ebook)
978-1-988824-72-7 (audiobook)

Front cover photograph of Eugene Stickland by Bart Habermiller.

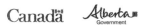

Durvile Publications would like to acknowledge the financial support of
the Government of Canada through the Canadian Heritage Canada Book Fund
and the Government of Alberta, Alberta Media Fund.
Printed in Canada. First edition, first printing. 2021.

Durvile Publications recognizes the traditional territories upon which our studios rest.
The Indigenous Peoples of Southern Alberta include the
Siksika, Piikani, and Kainai of the Blackfoot Confederacy; the Dene Tsuut'ina;
the Chiniki, Bearspaw, and Wesley Stoney Nakoda First Nations;
and the Region 3 Métis Nation of Alberta.

For Hanna

CONTENTS

—~m~—

—~m~—

CONTENTS

—w—

—w—

PREFACE

—꘭—

Isn't it funny how it works out? I never set out to
write medically themed plays, let alone three of them
and I would never have envisioned a book such as this
as part of my *oeuvre*, but here it is. And here you are
holding the book in your hands reading these words.
And so what can I assume about you, dear reader?
Maybe you are a student of some aspect of drama, or
theatre? Or maybe you are in the medical profession in
some way? Or maybe you are a fundraiser? Or someone whose life has been touched by one of the conditions I explore in these plays? Or perhaps someone you
love has had to deal with one of these afflictions? There
are so many possibilities. Clearly, this book is meant
to serve a lot of masters, as they say. I hope that I have
done a good job, and that you find something of value
in these pages, whatever your reason for being here.

As I say, I never set out to be a chronicler of medical conditions or syndromes or diseases, let alone in
the theatre, it just worked out that way. The first play
in this collection, *Closer and Closer Apart*, came about
as a result of my having read John Bayley's touching
memoir *Elegy for Iris* in which he chronicles his wife
Iris Murdoch's harrowing end of life experience with
Alzheimer disease. (In fact, I think it's quite possible that I stole the title of my play from a line in Mr.
Bayley's book. *C'est la guerre*, as they say. Talent bor-
rows, genius steals.)

Looking back (through Google, *etc.*) Mr. Bayley's book came out in 1999 and my play opened in 1999. That means reading his book must have had a profound and immediate effect on me. In 1999, my own mother was 80 years old and was in quite good health so the play was not based on any first-hand experience, purely a work of dramatic fiction. Sadly, the play was perhaps somewhat prescient as my mother was hit hard by Alzheimer several years later which was obviously a tremendously difficult ordeal for all of us in the family to go through. She also suffered from rheumatoid arthritis

—⁓—

I did what all writers do.
I made it up.
I used my imagination.

—⁓—

and sadly died in a great deal of pain and confusion. She was a good mother, a good person. I thought she deserved a better end than that, but isn't that the way with our reaction to all of these diseases?

I hardly knew what was to come when I wrote the play, so I did what all writers do in such a situation: I made it up. I used my imagination. I used Joe's monologues to hint at the brilliant sensitive mind lurking beneath the surface of his confusion. Perhaps that was being falsely optimistic. But this is a play, not a case study, and in the theatre people like to be entertained. Liberties are sometimes taken in the name of entertainment.

Closer and Closer Apart was first produced at Lunchbox Theatre in Calgary for a very appreciative audience. It was produced again for a small tour in Calgary as part of the Alberta 2005 celebrations marking the province's hundred-year anniversary as a Canadian province. The last stop on that mini tour was at an event called Alzheimer Awareness Week at the Hotchkiss Brain Institute at the University of Calgary. Our audience that night was comprised of researchers, doctors, nurses, caregivers, therapists, and family members of people with Alzheimer disease. The play proved to be a good place to start an in-depth examination of all aspects of the disease, from many different angles. But it was not expected to have been an accurate case study.

It's of interest to note, I believe, that *Closer and Closer Apart* was one of the first of many plays about Alzheimer disease to be written in Canada in the early years of this century. This for the simple reason that writers in the second wave of playwriting in Canada, of which I am a part, were experiencing Alzheimer disease up close and personally with their parents. My play may be unique in that it is a one act, with a playing time of just under an hour. A full-length version of the play was later written and performed at Theatre Network in Edmonton a few years after this one-act version received its premier production in Calgary in 2000. I was very proud of that production and I think I did a reasonable job of adapting my own work. And yet, the venerable Grant Reddick, who played Joe in the productions of the one-act version in Calgary, often refers to the one-act version as my "little gem" so we decided to include it in the current volume. I tend to think of it like a string quartet compared to my longer symphonic works.

Even at that, it is still the longest play in this collection. While *Closer and Closer Apart* was written for an actual theatre, the other two were written for special events — namely, fundraisers for research into their respective areas of concern, Stargardt disease and Parkinson disease. I am not a doctor or a researcher, but I did some reading and had the opportunity to talk with some experts in the field — enough to acquire the confidence needed to present these plays to audiences who knew a lot more about these afflictions than I ever will. Some of these experts have contributed essays to this book, for which I am extremely grateful.

Fade to Light was the first of these and it presented a unique theatrical opportunity. The fundraiser it was presented at was an ambitious affair held at Hotel Arts in downtown Calgary. Along with my play, attendees were served a full course meal with wine pairings — the catch was that you had to eat this meal blindfolded. (This was along the lines of the experience of diners at Noir Restaurant in Montreal. Did you know, for example, that even some experienced wine drinkers cannot distinguish a white from a red when blindfolded?) The dinner certainly demonstrated to us sighted people the importance of vision when it comes to eating — not only in terms of locating your food or glass of wine and getting it to your mouth, but in terms of taste as well.

Because of the unique nature of the evening, and having the audience blindfolded, I quickly realized that we could perform what is essentially a radio play, and so was able to set the play in the middle of a verdant park in the midst of a big city. I was able to call for a windstorm to shake the trees and a thunderstorm to roll in towards the end with lightning and lashing rains — all impossible effects to pull off on a make-shift stage in a hotel ballroom.

It led to one of my most cherished moments in my theatrical career — when the narrator began speaking, as one, the entire audience of a couple of hundred blind-folded people turned their heads towards the voice and craned their necks in such a way that they could hear better. This happened in one seemingly choreographed moment. It was as if the elite of Calgary society had been transformed into children waiting for their bedtime story. It was quite a sight for me to witness as I stood nervously at the back of the hall, silently cheering on my cast.

The final play in the collection, *The Last Dance,* was in support of technology being developed in Calgary and Beijing, China by Dr. Bin Hu. It is essentially a piece of equipment to help Parkinson patients improve their gait and thus reduce the chances of falling, which is a real and serious danger for people with the disease.

The idea for the play came to me under very sad circumstances. One day not long before I wrote the play, I received a friend request on Facebook from the woman whom I had dated off and on throughout high school. Her name was Debbie, and I hadn't talked to her probably since the night she dumped me at the grad prom (yes, she really did) some forty years earlier. She asked if I would mind her calling and I said of course not, and so we talked and the first thing she did was apologize for dumping me that night. I told her I had managed to get over it.

Then we got to the real reason for her call. She was dying. She had Amyotrophic Lateral Sclerosis (ALS, or Lou Gehrig's disease) and didn't have long to live. She wanted to say goodbye to me. I'm sure, dear reader, you can imagine the intensity and emotion of that call. I know a bit about ALS and what it does to the body. I wrote about it in *The Calgary Herald* years earlier. I edited and published the book *Cartwheels,* which is a collection of emails by Amy Doolittle from the last months of her life when she was dying from the same disease. When I was approached by the Branch Out Foundation to write a play having to do with Parkinson

—⚙—

Creating an event with a
play at its centre
makes for a memorable evening.

—⚙—

disease, I just took a few liberties and used my conversation with Debbie as the foundation for the play.

The Last Dance has a much longer run than *Fade to Light* — two nights! It was part of an event called *Your Brain on Art,* a fundraising event for the Branch Out Foundation in Calgary. This foundation is a fundraising organization that focuses on supporting research into the family of diseases including MS, ALS, Alzheimer, and Parkinson disease.

Taken all together, I believe they make an interesting collection, unique as far as I know in the annals of play publishing. It's always gratifying to have one's work published, let alone three at a time, and, on top of that, two very brief plays that I never imagined would be published in the first place.

I have seen all three plays produced for good reasons — to promote awareness of these various diseases, and to raise funds for research into each of them. In envisioning this volume, I had hopes that the plays might see the light of day, at least the lights of a stage, one more time, or maybe more. It's not that I have dreams of becoming rich from such productions — I know better than that by now. I believe creating an event with a play at its centre, whether for awareness or fund-generating for research, or both, truly makes for a memorable evening.

With this in mind, it is our hope (that is, my publisher's and my hope) that this volume will be of interest to people involved in theatre, especially those interested in playwriting, as well as fundraisers and people from the medical world.

A quick note about how we are referring to the diseases. Technically, in Canada, we do not add the apostrophe "s" after the names of eponymous diseases, so it is correct to say Alzheimer, Parkinson and Stargardt. Of course, no one says them this way in day-to-day life, including a world expert like Dr. Bin Hu in his essay. I am thankful to all the contributors who have provided their insights from their various perspectives.

All in all I hope we have created something special, with the whole being even greater than the sum of the parts.

> — *Eugene Stickland*
> *Calgary, Canada*
> *2021*

PART ONE

THE PLAYS

AND

COMMENTARIES

CLOSER AND CLOSER APART

A Play in One Act

by

Eugene Stickland

INTRODUCTION TO
CLOSER AND CLOSER APART

—॥॥—

STANDING AT NIGHT outside of McGiveny Hall on the St. Mary's University campus in south Calgary. I had just seen a performance of this play, *Closer and Closer Apart,* and another phenomenal performance by Grant Reddick in the role of Joe Ballantyne. I had come out for a quick smoke before going back in to handle a question and answer session. Then I heard a sound — someone crying. I looked along the back of the building, further into the shadows. Yes, there was a woman standing over there and she was crying. I approached warily.

As it turned out, we knew each other. We were not quite friends, but certainly warm acquaintances. I asked if she was alright. She told me her dad had had Alzheimer, and while she tried to be brave for the most part, the play had hit hard, devastating her. She didn't feel up to staying for the session. I helped her to her car and went back in.

Of course, you hope that your work touches people, moves them even. Yet I don't believe I'd ever seen it up close like that, so raw, and with someone I cared for. It touched me deeply, maybe even changed me to a certain extent. If, as artists, we are going to open wounds, touch nerves, we should do it as delicately and even as elegantly as possible. It is, I believe, an elegant play.

When I wrote it, there was only one person in our circle who had been known to suffer from Alzheimer. That was years ago when I still lived with my parents. The man in question was a former parish priest at our old church, St. Peter's Anglican. After retiring, he and his wife had moved to the country.

—ᴔ—

He had a faraway look in his eyes.
We didn't play the piano
together any longer.

—ᴔ—

They would visit from time to time — always unexpectedly and always at mealtime. (This was the way of country people at the time, I suppose. My mother never minded and always miraculously prepared enough food for everyone.) At that time, I was studying piano rather seriously, and the Good Father would from time to time drop in during the day with some piano music for four hands and we had a great time playing it. A lot of Haydn, I seem to recall.

But then things started to change. He might call and arrange to come over with some music but never show up. One night at dinner my mom reported that he had been discovered wandering around downtown, unable to locate his car. If he and his wife did drop in for dinner, something was clearly wrong. He had a faraway look in his eyes. We didn't play the piano together any longer. And as it does, it went from bad to worse.

He was the only one of my personal acquaintances who was thus afflicted. My grandma, my mom's mom, lived to be 101 and was sharp as a tack, as they say, right until the end. It was my mom who would end up with Alzheimer a few years after I wrote this play. It was not very pretty at the end. Fortunately, the research I had done for the play had included "how to be" around a loved one with the disease. I suppose I could say I transformed my frustration into compassion and we got by as well as we could. Still, it was a sad and difficult time.

One other thing comes to mind when I consider this play of mine written over twenty years ago now as I write this. I hadn't wanted to write it. I had just written five plays in five years for Alberta Theatre Projects. They had all done very well, very well-received. They were getting productions far and wide, winning awards. I was feeling a little burned out. Also, I was in my forties and thinking a change in life might be in order. I began to dream of going back to university and studying to become an architect. I began to read about buildings and the people who designed them. On a trip to New York around this time, posing as a Canadian architect, I was given a tour of the Seagram Building, Mies van der Rohe's majestic minimalist masterwork on Park Avenue. I was in heaven.

On returning to Calgary a few days later, I an-

announced the exciting news to my wife, Carrie. Something along the lines of, "Guess what, honey? I've decided to become an architect!" She asked me if I was crazy, mad, insane, off my rocker. She reminded me that I had just tossed off a string of hit plays and was getting more productions than anyone in the country. And had I lost my mind entirely!? Giving up a career most people would die for to go back to school for years so I could design strip malls?! *Etc. Etc. Etc.*

—◊—

He had a faraway look in his eyes.
We didn't play the piano
together any longer.

—◊—

Well, that didn't go so well. It went even worse when I announced my intention to my artistic partner, Bob White, the following evening. Bob had an alter ego known as Buzz, and it soon became apparent that it was Buzz, not Bob, I was addressing. Carrie had been at least somewhat understanding, Buzz a little less so, to put it mildly.

So much for the exciting career change. Maybe it was nothing more than a mid-life crisis. The good news was, I had gotten inside the mind of an architect and I'd done all kinds of reading on the subject, so there was no point in letting all that go for naught. I wrote the play and somehow satisfied my urge to contribute to the field of architecture effectively, killing two birds with one stone.

One final thought. While I was casting about and eyeing a career change, a friend put me in touch with an architect here in Calgary. He invited me up to his office and we had a good chat about theatre, architecture, and life in general. He counselled me that if you do the thing you really love for a living, it may lose some of its lustre, and become like any other job. You should try to do the thing you love second best for a living, and maintain your love for that other thing, keep it pure.

I thought that was very good advice.

CLOSER AND CLOSER APART

Closer and Closer Apart was first presented at the Lunchbox Theatre in Calgary, Alberta, opening October 18, 1999 with the following personnel:

Joe Ballantyne .... Grant Reddick
Melody Ballantyne................. Carrie Schiffler

Director................................... Bob White
Stage Manager........................ Sylvia Falez
Musical Director.................... Kevin McGugan
Set Design.............................. Witek Wisniewski

The play was commissioned by Lunchbox Theatre as part of the Petro-Canada Stage One Series.

Closer and Closer Apart

Characters

JOE BALLANTYNE, a retired architect, widowed some time in the past, now in the early stages of Alzheimer disease.

MELODY BALLANTYNE, his daughter, recently separated, stopping in on Joe en route to Chicago.

Setting

The living room of Joe's high rise condo/apartment, upscale and downtown. Simple yet extremely elegant and modern furnishings. The entire back wall is comprised of bookshelves, which start out orderly enough at the upper left hand corner, but fall into chaos as they go along. On the floor and on the tables and chairs, there are books and periodicals piled everywhere. Everything contributing to a sense of impending chaos. The downstage view would be of a city skyline.

Time

The action of the play takes place in our own time, over the course of a few days.

Scene One

> *Lights up. Morning. JOE is sitting in a chair, covered with books and periodicals. He reads for a few moments, then seems to drift off into sleep. He comes to, then rises from his chair. The books spill off his lap. He yawns and stretches. He picks up one of the books from the floor —* Gray's Anatomy *— and crosses to the bookcase. He finds the place where the book should go, is about to put it in place, then seems to lose his will to do so. He lets the book drop to the floor and exits. Blackout.*

End of Scene

—⁓—

Scene Two

> *Lights up on the living room, empty. After a moment JOE enters and goes to the bookcase, to the place where he started to shelve his copy of* Gray's Anatomy. *He pulls out a few books, but obviously he can't find it. He puts on an overcoat and leaves. Blackout.*

End of Scene

—⁓—

Scene Three

Lights up. A little later. MELODY enters the apartment, carrying a carry-on bag and a laptop computer. She is well dressed. She takes in the apartment for a moment, picks up a few books, including Gray's Anatomy, *and starts reshelving them. She suddenly stops. She backs away from the shelves, clearly intending to avoid any filing away of the books. As she is doing this, JOE enters, still in his coat, holding a bookstore bag. She turns and sees him.*

JOE: Who are you?!

Blackout.

End of Scene

Scene Four

> *Lights up. JOE is sitting in his chair
> again. He glances towards the kitchen,
> nervously. He picks up his bag, takes out
> a brand new copy of* Gray's Anatomy,
> *begins to read, realizes he doesn't have
> his glasses. He gropes around under the
> books and magazines, then suddenly
> remembers they are pushed up on his
> head. He slides them down into position.
> MELODY enters with a cup of cocoa for
> each of them.*

MELODY: There you go.
JOE: Thank you ...
MELODY: Just the way you like it.
JOE: Mmmmm ...
MELODY: With marshmallows.
JOE: Ah yes ...
MELODY: That's still how you like it, isn't it?
JOE: I think so.
MELODY: It used to be.
JOE: Yes ...

> *Slight pause. They sip their cocoa.*

MELODY: How is it?
JOE: It's good.
MELODY: That's good.
JOE: Is it Fry's?
MELODY: Yeah.
JOE: It's good.

MELODY:	Good ... anything else I can get for you?
JOE:	No ... that's OK. This is good.
MELODY:	Good.
JOE:	It's Fry's?
MELODY:	Yes. It's Fry's.
JOE:	That's good.
MELODY:	Yeah ... It's good ... Everything's good ...

They sip their cocoa.

MELODY:	It's so good to see you again.
JOE:	Yes ...
MELODY:	I guess I startled you. Sorry. I know it's been a while ...
JOE:	Just wasn't expecting to find anyone here ...
MELODY:	That's why I called.
JOE:	That's right ...
MELODY:	You hadn't forgotten that I called.
JOE:	No, no. It just may have slipped my mind ... you know.
MELODY:	Yeah. I know what it's like. It happens to me all the time .... Anyway it all worked out to stop in for a few days. Got the flights and the stopover. I thought I'll look in on you. Tell you myself.
JOE:	Tell me what?
MELODY:	About the Chicago thing. And about Charles ...
JOE:	Oh yeah.
MELODY:	Yeah ...
JOE:	Charlie ...
MELODY:	Yeah. Funny how it turned out that everything you said about him was right.

JOE:	He was boring.
MELODY:	Yeah.
JOE:	Tedious.
MELODY:	I know.
JOE:	And I always thought there was something strange going on with his eyes. They were set too close together. Some inbreeding going on there or something. I found it very hard to be in the same room as him.
MELODY:	Yeah yeah. Let's move on, OK Dad?
JOE:	OK.
MELODY:	So, yeah, anyway ... Like I said, it seemed like a good time to cut my losses and move on. It's a good opportunity.
JOE:	What is it again?
MELODY:	What is what?
JOE:	The opportunity.
MELODY:	I just told you. Ten minutes ago.
JOE:	Right, right. Uh ...
MELODY:	Chicago.
JOE:	Right. Chicago. I was there.
MELODY:	I know. I remember that.
JOE:	I gave a paper.
MELODY:	I know you did.
JOE:	I met Mies van der Rohe. That was quite a thrill ...
MELODY:	I remember ...
JOE:	You weren't even born.
MELODY:	It's part of the family mythology.
JOE:	Of course ... "God is in the details ...." He said that, you know.
MELODY:	Yeah.

JOE: He didn't say it to me, but he supposedly said it.

MELODY: Right.

JOE: He also said "Less is more." Again, not to me .... And I'm not sure that I agree with that. But I do agree that God is, in fact, in the details.

MELODY: Absolutely.

JOE: Wouldn't that be something ... ? When you're gone, to have said one perfect thing that everyone would remember. Like Mies van der Rohe. "God is in the details ... " A measurement of yourself in words. I'm not sure that I've ever said anything that profound, or simple, or both. Ah well ... That was a long time ago. Chicago ... the windy city. That's what they call it. And they're right about that. It's very windy. Right by the lake.... You'll need to take a scarf or something for your hair ...

MELODY: Right.

Slight pause.

JOE: This is good cocoa.

MELODY: Good.

JOE: Just how I like it

MELODY: I know ...

Slight pause.

JOE: I uh — ...

MELODY: What?

JOE: This thing in Chicago.

MELODY: Yeah?

JOE:	What you're doing?
MELODY:	Yeah?
JOE:	I'm not sure I get it.
MELODY:	What's to get?
JOE:	What do you call it again?
MELODY:	Head hunting.
JOE:	Head hunting. Right. I'm not sure I get it.
MELODY:	I know it's not what you saw me doing for a living. And you know, I tried design school and that didn't work out. There's nothing I can do about that now. I guess I'm attracted to the idea of moving people's lives around. And I don't mind the money, either. I don't think there's anything wrong with it.
JOE:	With what?
MELODY:	With what I do for a living.
JOE:	I'm not saying there's anything wrong with it dear.
MELODY:	What are you saying?
JOE:	I'm saying I don't fully understand what it is.
MELODY:	Ohhhh ... Head hunting? Personnel reallocation?
JOE:	I'm still not clear ...
MELODY:	Remember that time we almost moved to Montreal. Because someone had offered you a new job. A better job? I was about ten.
JOE:	Ahhhh ....That's what you do?
MELODY:	Yeah.
JOE:	People shouldn't leave their provinces. Or even their home towns, for that matter. Maybe for college. Or a war or something like that. *(Indicating the window)* You look out there, these days it's all people from Saskatchewan.

	Why don't they just go back home? You can't even find a parking spot downtown anymore. I mean, really. It's too much ...
MELODY:	That's all you have to say about it?
JOE:	And just to warn you: you'll always be a stranger in a city you didn't grow up in.
MELODY:	Yeah, OK. You don't think people should move around, that's your opinion. It's not what I think. I think I like Chicago. I'm looking forward to it. I don't care what you say. It'll be good to get away for a while .... Actually, I do care what you say, but I'm definitely going. So maybe don't say anything else, OK?
JOE:	OK.
MELODY:	OK. Thanks

Pause. She looks around the room, goes to the book case and picks up the copy of Gray's Anatomy *from the floor.*

	I can't believe the state of your books, dad.
JOE:	I know. It's a disgrace.
MELODY:	It never got like this when I was at home.
JOE:	You think this is bad. You should see the periodicals ...
MELODY:	Bad?
JOE:	Out of control.
MELODY:	People don't believe me when I tell them you taught me to read and write when I was only three so I could do your filing for you.
JOE:	Most people don't really understand filing, when you get right down to it.
MELODY:	*(Holding up the book)* You've been reading Gray's Anatomy?

JOE: (*Suddenly aware that he's holding another copy of the same book, and hiding it from her*) I'm always reading it.

MELODY: Why?

JOE: I like the idea of folding back the skin and seeing what's underneath ... all those hidden things we try not to think about ...

MELODY: Whatever .... Do you want me to put it back, or what? Man. There I go. I'm doing it. I walked in and I saw the shelf and right away, I thought I have to get everything back into order. But I'm not doing it. You can do it. There's nothing wrong with you. You're mobile. I've got too much on my mind to get your books back in order. It can just stay here on the floor.

> *She puts the book down on the floor, returns to her chair and sits down. They both look at the book, and at each other, and at the book. After a moment, she gets back up and picks up the book. She goes to the shelf.*

MELODY: (*Referring to the system of cataloguing*) What is this system, Dad?

JOE: Dewey. What do you think?

MELODY: It looks pretty much random to me.

JOE: It's in need of some serious maintenance.

MELODY: I'll say .... So where does Gray's Anatomy go?

JOE: You don't remember?

MELODY: No.

JOE: Come on.

MELODY: I don't.

29

JOE:	You used to know the Dewey Decimal System inside out. I can't believe you'd just forget it.
MELODY:	I know it's hard to believe —
JOE:	All those hours we spent —
MELODY:	Oh yeah. I remember all those hours —
JOE:	I can't believe you'd just forget the whole system.
MELODY:	That was years ago.
JOE:	Think!
MELODY:	Oh brother. OK. Let me see ... 600's, I guess.
JOE:	Close ...
MELODY:	610? No. 611. God help me. I do remember it. 611. I can't believe this. Brother, I said I wouldn't do this and here I am. 611 .... *(She puts the book back)* It hardly matters anyway, your system is in such a mess. Anyway. There we go. Back on the shelf. Safe and sound.

Slight pause.

JOE:	You don't have to worry about it, you know. If it still bothers you.
MELODY:	No?
JOE:	It will all get organized, when Mrs. Hauser gets back.
MELODY:	Mrs. Hauser?
JOE:	Yeah.
MELODY:	What are you talking about?
JOE:	She's let things slide a bit, but it won't take her long to get everything back into apple pie order.
MELODY:	You think Mrs. Hauser's going to do something about these books for you?
JOE:	Of course. When she gets back.

MELODY: Back? From where?

JOE: From wherever she is.

MELODY: Where do you think she is?

JOE: I don't know.

MELODY: When was the last time you saw her?

JOE: I can't remember.

MELODY: Roughly.

JOE: I don't know.

MELODY: Ball park.

JOE: I'm not sure.

MELODY: Give or take a month. Or a year. When do you think you saw her last?

JOE: I don't know.

MELODY: Think!

JOE: I am thinking! What do you think I'm doing? I'm thinking! What was I ... ?

MELODY: Mrs. Hauser.

JOE: Mrs. Hauser. Right. She'll come. She always comes. Every Tuesday. Maybe there's something the matter with Dennis, I don't know. Or the cat or something.

MELODY: Dog.

JOE: There's no dog.

MELODY: There's a dog — There was a dog. There was no cat. She couldn't stand cats.

JOE: How am I supposed to know? I can't be expected to keep track of her every movement.

MELODY: Actually, Dad, keeping track of Mrs. Hauser's every movement for the last ten years or so wouldn't really be all that difficult.

JOE: No?

MELODY:	No.
JOE:	Why's that?
MELODY:	Because she's dead.
JOE:	She is?
MELODY:	Yes.
JOE:	Mrs. — ?
MELODY:	Mrs. Hauser.
JOE:	Dead?
MELODY:	Yes.
JOE:	No she's not.
MELODY:	Yes she is.
JOE:	She's old. I'll give you that. She's not in the best of shape — that terrible thing with her knees and all. And those horrible shoes she has to wear. But she's not dead.
MELODY:	We went to her funeral.
JOE:	I don't think so.
MELODY:	You delivered her eulogy. You talked for thirty minutes about her innate understanding of the Dewey Decimal System. There wasn't a dry eye in the church. Of course there wasn't a dry eye, they were all librarians. You started a scholarship at the university in her name. For God's sake, Dad. You have to remember this!
JOE:	It was raining ... ?
MELODY:	Yes.
JOE:	And someone had a flat tire at the cemetery.
MELODY:	Uncle Frank.
JOE:	Ah yes ...
MELODY:	You remember?
JOE:	Yes ... poor Mrs. Hauser. She was a fine, fine librarian. What a tragic loss.

Lights change. JOE crosses the stage and picks up his new copy of Gray's Anatomy *from his chair. He opens it, and speaks directly to the audience.*

JOE: Page 691 of Gray's Anatomy. There is a diagrammatic representation of the cells of the cerebellum. It's a strange looking drawing. If you hadn't found it in Gray's Anatomy, if you'd simply come across it with no idea of its context, you might well believe it was the diagrammatic representation of petroglyphs — like those carved by the Plains Indians in ancient times. Strange creatures with a single eye at their centre, many tentacles radiating outward, all seemingly engaged in some kind of ritual — searching perhaps for some kind of shelter, or sanity ... some sense of place and well-being in the uncaring world around them. Perhaps the first impulse toward mythology ... religion. Over the years, the petroglyphs have been worn away by the elements, until only the faintest impression is left ... and all the depth and detail and meaning have all but vanished without a trace ... like the writing on the mind, the memories that fade with the passing years, and finally all that is left is a smooth face of stone, revealing nothing as we finally forget even ourselves ...

Blackout.

End of Scene

—∞—

Scene Five

> *Lights up. MELODY is trying to make sense of some of the books, putting a few of them back on the shelves. JOE is in his chair, reading* Gray's Anatomy.

MELODY: It's funny, I guess. Not really. I know I don't write that much. That's just me. Not how I feel about you. I just assumed that you were OK here. You've got your books, your periodicals. Didn't you have a little something to do a while back? A chapel or something? Wasn't there some kind of contract?

JOE: It was a sculptor. Studio, gallery. One of those flaky middle aged guys with the beard ... and dust everywhere ...

MELODY: How did that go?

JOE: It was OK.

MELODY: Just OK?

JOE: Well, you know ...

MELODY: No, I don't know. That's why I'm asking.

JOE: It was going fine, at first. I know how those people are. Expose the beams. Natural materials. Let in the light. No big mystery. And it was going well enough. It was really a design job. They didn't need me. They needed a designer. Which I can do. But it felt good, so I played along ...

MELODY: So what happened?

JOE: You don't really want to know.

MELODY: Yeah, I do.

JOE: Well ... I was OK here, doing the drawings. Talking on the phone. Things were moving

along. I was doing OK. But then one day, I had
to go there, to the site. No big deal, right? I got
dressed. I got in the car. I was going there. I
was in my car. But I couldn't find it. The site.
I didn't know which way, which direction. I
didn't even know what it looked like. It was
my design, my building, and I could have
driven right by it. And not even seen it. In
fact, I probably did drive right by it. I didn't
have a clue .... And this feeling of being lost
and disoriented is all coming on while I'm
behind the wheel of the car. And all of the
sudden, I looked in the rear view mirror, and
there's this old man in the mirror, leering at
me, squinched up over seat, this old grey man,
and he put his hands out and grabbed me
by the throat, choking me. I couldn't see the
road. I couldn't breathe. And he had me by the
throat and he was choking me and he's saying,
"You lost it Joe ... it's gone. Go home. Just go
home ... Just go home .... " But I couldn't even
get back home on my own. They had to bring
me home. I didn't even know where I was
anymore .... I haven't been in that car since. In
fact, you can have the car. It probably needs an
oil change by now, but you can have it. I take
cabs these days. Anyway, I had to give it up.
The job. I passed it over to one of the younger
designers. No big deal.

MELODY:	Well ...
JOE:	Yeah. I'm sorry ...
MELODY:	What are you sorry about?
JOE:	I don't want to be a bother, you know ... I wouldn't have bothered you, or Michael, or anyone —

MELODY:	Have you seen Michael?
JOE:	No, I don't see him. He has his own family now. He's busy. I manage quite well on my own. Until this business in the car. I wouldn't have said anything, but you showed up. It's very hard to hide this. I mean, look. *(Holding up a little notebook)* I've got notes. *(Reading)* "Melody. Daughter. Mother deceased. Separated from Charlie. Boring husband." *(Not reading)* Without my notes, it can be very hard to make the connections. Everything just starts moving too fast or something ... I get extremely confused. Obviously, Melody, something is happening to me ...
MELODY:	You have to remind yourself that Mom's dead?
JOE:	I have trouble remembering her at all ...
MELODY:	Oh ...
JOE:	I've tried that thing they're talking about ... you know ... the herbal thing—
MELODY:	Gingko?
JOE:	Yeah.
MELODY:	Did it help?
JOE:	I don't know. I can never remember whether I've taken it or not.
MELODY:	Really?
JOE:	No, I'm joking.
MELODY:	Oh.
JOE:	I think it helped for a while .... But it's no kind of cure.
MELODY:	What does your doctor say?
JOE:	He quit.
MELODY:	What do you mean he quit?

JOE:	He just up and quit. He wrote a nice letter to all his patients and said good luck and he quit. He's painting now in BC or some such thing.
MELODY:	What do you mean?
JOE:	They do this calender every year. They have art work by physicians on it. He got a painting on the calender a few years ago and it went to his head. Now he thinks he's an artist. He's lost his perspective.
MELODY:	There's other doctors.
JOE:	I don't know them.
MELODY:	Get to know them.
JOE:	They don't know me.
MELODY:	Well, you've got to go to someone, Dad. I mean, little old men in your car trying to strangle you? That's not a healthy thing. That's not normal. You need a doctor. I'll help you find one.
JOE:	No.
MELODY:	Yes.
JOE:	Listen. I know what's going on. I'm not stupid. I know my mind, and what it's doing. I've lived inside this mind all my life. But the trouble is, you start going to doctors, they start naming things. You know what I'm saying. They start looking in that blue book of theirs and you're done for.
MELODY:	I don't know if that's such a bad thing.
JOE:	It's a terrible thing.
MELODY:	Why?
JOE:	They name it. They pretend they can fix it. They take you away from what you know ... from your books and your view and you end

up being this messy grey shuffling thing groping your way down a hallway ... and they treat you like you're some kind of hero when you manage to take a piss in the morning ... in the toilet. I'm not ... I'm not prepared to go there. I'll stay here. And if I have to use my last ounce of rational thought to throw myself out that window, I'll be happy. Because if I'm going to vacate my brain, then what's left? You tell me what's left. You find a doctor who can look in his blue book and who can tell me what's left.

MELODY: But there's cures, Dad.

JOE: There's no cures.

MELODY: There's medication. There's stuff you can take, stuff you can do—

JOE: Is there?

MELODY: There's got to be.

JOE: You think I haven't read on this? You think I just go willingly into all of this? No way. I've done the reading. This, this, this dried up leaf—

MELODY: Gingko —

JOE: It's not hurting. But it's not the answer either.

MELODY: Jeez ...

JOE: What?

MELODY: How am I supposed to go away, with all this happening?

JOE: You call a cab. You go to the airport. You say goodbye. You fly away. It's easy.

MELODY: I can't just leave you like this.

JOE: Yes you can.

MELODY: No I can't.

JOE: I didn't ask you to come back. I'm not asking you to stay.

MELODY: But I can't just go.

JOE: Oh yes you can. Whatever will happen to me will happen to me with or without you here. It's got nothing to do with you.

Slight pause.

MELODY: Well, that's just it right there, isn't it Dad?

JOE: What?

MELODY: You don't think that I could make any difference to your life. All I'm capable of is clipping articles from your magazines and filing them away for you. Keeping your bookcase in order. But you've never actually thought that I could make any difference.

JOE: That's not true.

MELODY: Really?

JOE: Not at all. Of course you make a difference to my life —

MELODY: How?

JOE: I don't know. By being who you are?

MELODY: Who do you think I am?

JOE: You're my daughter.

MELODY: Who does your filing. Who puts your books on the shelf.

JOE: It's more than that.

MELODY: Yeah? What?

JOE: Listen, darling. I look out this window every day; it's like looking at my portfolio or something. All those buildings of mine, and my friends. I seemed to have had a hand in most of them. I was a part of the movement that created them. Wouldn't you think I'd get some measure of satisfaction from looking out there? Some sense of accomplishment? Well, I don't. All I see is failure. I see the flaws. All that cold glass, reflecting straight lines. There's no beauty that I see, or feel, out there. Just cold function. Strain. Stress. Failure. But when I look at you, I see the one worthwhile creation of my life — well, at least something that I had a hand in. I don't see any flaws. Maybe they're there. Maybe you see them when you look in the mirror at yourself. I don't see them, or if I do, I guess I just don't care. I see only a beautiful young woman. It's only through you that I feel there's any redemption to my life. The rest simply doesn't matter.

MELODY: Wow .... Really?

JOE: Yeah. I'm very proud of you.

MELODY: Oh yeah?

JOE: Yeah .... And I want you to get on with your life.

MELODY: I don't know ...

JOE: I'm asking you, Melody. Please. Go to Chicago. Don't waste this opportunity here with me. No one can change anything here ...

MELODY: OK.

JOE: Promise?

MELODY: Yeah.

JOE: OK. Well .... That's enough for me. That's all I can do, to do what I just did. To hold it together to have any kind of conversation. It exhausts me. I'm sorry. I need to lie down.

MELODY: Sure.

JOE:	*(Starting to leave)* I'm glad you came.
MELODY:	Yeah. Me too.
JOE:	*(Starting to leave again)* Oh. And there's something else ...
MELODY:	What?
JOE:	I love you.
MELODY:	Yeah?
JOE:	Yeah.
MELODY:	Thanks.
JOE:	You're welcome ...
MELODY:	You go rest. I'll get something started for dinner.

He doesn't go, but stands there,
staring at her.

MELODY:	What?
JOE:	Jeez, it's no wonder it didn't work out with you and what's his name ...
MELODY:	What?
JOE:	Someone says I love you, you say it back. Even if you don't necessarily mean it. Or if it's uncomfortable to say, for whatever reason. You say it. I thought I taught you that.
MELODY:	You did.
JOE:	Right. So ... ?
MELODY:	I love you, Dad.
JOE:	That's my girl. OK. That's enough of that stuff. I'm going to lie down. See you later.

He leaves. Fade on MELODY to blackout.

End of Scene

Scene Six

> *Lights up on JOE. He is sitting in the*
> *middle of the living room floor with a*
> *big pile of* Architectural Reviews *and a*
> *pair of scissors. MELODY enters from*
> *her room, carrying her bag and laptop*
> *computer.*

MELODY: Well, I think I got everything. I guess you can always send anything — What are you doing?

JOE: What?

MELODY: What are you doing with those?

JOE: There was an article I think I must have read ... once upon a time ... that must have been about something ... that I thought I needed to know. And I feel if I could only find it, and clip it, and start a folder for it, and file it ... then I would recognize it, and then I would know what it is that I think I need to know ... that I don't know ... now ...

MELODY: Right ...

JOE: I don't know what it is, so it's hard to find. But I'll know it when I see it. I think. I believe. And then ... I'll surely know. What was his name again?

MELODY: Who?

JOE: The man I'm looking for. Whose article I need to cut. And file. And paste. So I'll know ...

MELODY: I don't know.

JOE: No ... No one knows ...

> *Slight pause.*

JOE:	Where is it again?
MELODY:	What?
JOE:	The place you're going?
MELODY:	Chicago.
JOE:	Right ... That's right. I remember. I was there ... I gave a paper.
MELODY:	I know.
JOE:	I was there and I met ... uh, what's his name? God is in the Seagram Building ...
MELODY:	Mies van der Rohe.
JOE:	That's right ... That's it! That's who I'm looking for. *(Pointing to the magazines with his scissors)* He's in here somewhere!
MELODY:	I'm sure he is.
JOE:	Chicago. You see it all comes together in plain forms and sumptuous materials — of course more in New York where I didn't give a paper. Tough town.
MELODY:	Oh yeah?
JOE:	Nasty town.
MELODY:	New York or Chicago?
JOE:	Chicago. It's the kind of town where they kill you, just for crossing the street. You go left, when you should have gone right. You're bound to encounter someone who doesn't have your best interests at heart. It happened to a friend of mine ... ended up a couple of blocks the other side of some street no one crosses and that was it for him. They sent him home in plastic bags. One for his head — the other for what was left of him. That's Chicago. Even New York's not that bad. Or is it? The will of an epoch translated into

space. I find that more in New York, hardly here at all. What is the will here? What is the translation? We have the space. I never should have worked here, spent my life here. Nothing interesting happens when you have too much space. Anyway, that whole country is rotten to the core. I would be extremely cautious if I were you. They drop bombs on people halfway across the world just so they can have their freshly squeezed orange juice in the morning ... Which reminds me ...

Pause. She sets down her suitcase and computer.

MELODY:	Oh boy.
JOE:	What?
MELODY:	Nothing. I gotta tell you, Dad, I don't quite know what to do here.
JOE:	Do you not?
MELODY:	No.
JOE:	Why is that?
MELODY:	Well, yesterday, you asked me to go ...
JOE:	Yes ...
MELODY:	You made me promise to go ...
JOE:	Yes ...
MELODY:	And now I'm not so sure it's such a good idea.
JOE:	No?
MELODY:	No.
JOE:	I see ... Tell me ....
MELODY:	Yes?
JOE:	Is it the filing you're worried about? The clipping? Does it seem too much?

MELODY:	No, it's not that.
JOE:	Because Mrs. Hauser can easily handle this pile. She's very capable.
MELODY:	If she gets here ...
JOE:	Oh, she'll come. She very dependable ...

Slight pause.

MELODY:	I could help you find it ... I guess ...
JOE:	Find what?
MELODY:	The article you're looking for.
JOE:	Oh yes ...
MELODY:	On Mies van der Rohe, right?
JOE:	Yes, I think that's right.
MELODY:	*(Indicating the magazines)* Have you gone through any of these?
JOE:	I don't think so.
MELODY:	I'll help you, OK?
JOE:	That'd be great.
MELODY:	OK. Let's have a look, and see what we can find ...

She sits down on the floor beside JOE. Together they start going through the first magazine. Blackout.

End of Scene

—ww—

Scene Seven

> *The next day. Lights up on MELODY who is on the floor, going through the growing pile of* Architectural Reviews. *JOE appears with a rolled up towel.*

JOE: You're still here?

MELODY: Yeah.

JOE: I thought we talked about that.

MELODY: We did.

JOE: Well?

MELODY: I don't believe we decided on anything.

JOE: No, I guess we didn't .... I realize that yesterday I was not perhaps crystal clear in some of my processes.

MELODY: You know that, do you?

JOE: Yes. And I've been thinking about it.

MELODY: Yeah?

JOE: I was thinking that maybe you could help me.

MELODY: That's why I'm still here.

JOE: Good. So, I was reading this article.

MELODY: Oh yeah ...

JOE: In of those cheap publications one finds in the racks at a coffee shop. You know the ones .... You've seen them?

MELODY: Yes.

JOE: I read this article in a publication devoted to health. Actually, it even went beyond the concept of health into an area they refer to as — Oh brother. What was it again ... ?

MELODY: Wellness?

JOE: What the hell is that?

MELODY: I don't know. It's like health, I guess. Only more so. Kind of a lifestyle thing.

JOE: That's ludicrous. That's not even a word. But that wouldn't stop them trading on it .... No, it definitely wasn't wellness. Oh brother. Health and ... health and ....

MELODY: Fitness?

JOE: That's it.

MELODY: Physical fitness.

JOE: Right. Health and fitness ...

MELODY: OK. And so ...

JOE: What?

MELODY: You read an article on health and fitness ...

JOE: Right. Right ... Now, bear in mind, I'm not naming anything here ...

MELODY: No ...

JOE: The notion behind this article seemed to be that a certain amount of intense physical movement, might, by stimulating the flow of blood to certain areas of the body — for example, the brain — might — they say might — help alleviate certain symptoms of certain unnamed conditions. What do you think?

MELODY: Sounds plausible.

JOE: Now, you may recall as a part of our own family mythology that I once quarterbacked my high school football team to a Division B Championship.

MELODY: I've seen the trophy.

JOE: Right. I only mention this to make the point that my athletic prowess has clearly been established, although, admittedly, I may have

	backed off a bit from such pursuits these past 40 or 50 years. I certainly don't see myself joining up with some old timers football team, if such a thing even exists, and certainly my knees wouldn't hold up — you may recall I suffered damage to the anterior cruciate ligament of my left knee when I slipped on some scaffolding at a construction site a few years back.
MELODY:	Oh yeah.
JOE:	You remember that, do you?
MELODY:	I'd say your left knee is also a part of the family mythology, Dad.
JOE:	Right.
MELODY:	In fact, I remember Mom saying, "If I have to hear about that bloody knee of yours one more time I'm going to jump off a bridge."
JOE:	Yeah yeah yeah. Whatever. The point I'm trying to make is that I believe there is a certain amount of sagacity in this article which I read — and which I clipped, by the way, and which we'll need to file, although I have no category for health and uh, fitness, so we'll have to make one.
MELODY:	A category.
JOE:	That's right.
MELODY:	OK.
JOE:	Great ...

Slight pause.

| MELODY: | So what's with the towel, Dad? |
| JOE: | Hmmm? |

MELODY: What's with the towel?

JOE: *(Suddenly remembering that he's got the towel)* Oh. Yes. Of course. This is the point of what we've been talking about, isn't it?

MELODY: Is it?

JOE: Absolutely. Because as I say, I don't see myself jumping back onto the gridiron. So, instead, I am going to pursue something I was very good at, as a child, but that I haven't done for probably fifty years. Voila!

He unfolds the towel to reveal an extremely skimpy Speedo swim suit.

JOE: Swimming.

MELODY: You're going to wear that thing?

JOE: Yeah.

MELODY: In public?

JOE: Well, I'll be in the pool. Why? Is there something wrong with it?

MELODY: Seems a tad skimpy, don't you think?

JOE: That's what I used to say about some of the outfits you used to parade around in, but no one's going to be looking at this old body anyway so what difference does it make?

MELODY: You're probably right.

JOE: So what do you think?

MELODY: I think it's great.

JOE: Do you think?

MELODY: Yes. A bit of exercise. It can't hurt anything.

JOE: That's what I thought.

Slight pause.

JOE:	So ... have you seen my new car?
MELODY:	No.
JOE:	You're going to like it. It's a beemer. Rag top. Very fast car .... Like I say, you're welcome to it. Would you like to see it?
MELODY:	Sure.
JOE:	Maybe go for a little drive? To the pool? So I can have my swim.
MELODY:	You mean right now?
JOE:	Well, that's why I'm holding my trunks and my towel.
MELODY:	Do you have the keys?
JOE:	They should be on the little thingy in the hall.
MELODY:	Great. Let's go to the pool then. I'll find the keys.

She leaves. Lights change. JOE speaks directly to the audience.

JOE: At its best, architecture provides the illusion that we are not reaching up from the ground, but that rather that we have been suspended from the sky. Hovering in a crystal clear solution, floating between heaven and earth. And so we travel back to the sensation of our original dwelling place on the earth, when we were surrounded and protected in the dark rhythmic water, blissfully ignorant of ourselves and our place in the world ...

He leaves. Blackout.

End of Scene

Scene Eight

> *In blackout, the sound of shattering glass, very loud.*

End of Scene

—∿—

Scene Nine

> *Lights up. JOE is sitting in his chair, drinking a mug of cocoa. MELODY is pacing in front of him.*

MELODY: How's your cocoa?
JOE: Good. Is it Fry's?
MELODY: Yeah.
JOE: It's good.
MELODY: Good ... anything else I can get for you?
JOE: No ... that's OK. This is good.
MELODY: Good.

> *Slight pause.*

JOE: It's Fry's?
MELODY: Yes, Dad. It's Fry's.
JOE: That's good.
MELODY: Yeah .... It's good .... Everything's good ...

> *Pause.*

MELODY: I don't know what to say, Dad.
JOE: No.

Eugene Stickland

MELODY: I just don't know. I know we're not naming anything here—

JOE: No, we're not.

MELODY: But I think we're just kidding ourselves that things will get any better without some help. I mean, the pool and swimming and all that, it seemed like a good idea. But when you start smashing mirrors in the change room, then I can't help but think what we're doing isn't working. And even if it means naming it, and finding something to take, I think we need to think about doing that. Find something that's better for you, in the long run .... You know?

Pause.

JOE: It is Fry's?

MELODY: YES IT'S FUCKING FRY'S!! Sorry, Dad. Sorry. I didn't mean to. Sorry ...

JOE: It's good.

MELODY: Good. I'm sorry. I didn't mean to raise my voice. I just don't understand why you smashed that mirror with a chair at the pool. What was going through your head?

JOE: I saw him.

MELODY: Who?

JOE: The guy.

MELODY: What guy?

JOE: The guy who's been following me. The guy who was in my car that time. He was there. I thought I could nail him with the chair. But obviously he got away ...

MELODY: I see ...

JOE: He's extremely elusive.

MELODY: Yes. I guess he is ...

> *Slight pause.*

MELODY: How's your cocoa?
JOE: All gone. It was good. Can I have some more?
MELODY: No. I want you to go lie down for a while. We've had a rich, full day and you need to get some rest. OK?
JOE: OK ...
MELODY: I'll see you later.
JOE: OK.

> *He leaves for his bedroom. Lights fade on MELODY. Blackout.*

End of Scene

—⚮—

Scene Ten

> *Lights up on Melody, talking on the phone.*

MELODY: Yeah. Yeah. Yeah. I know. Yeah. Well, he's your father too, Michael. Yeah, I know how busy you are. Oh, I know. Listen. Listen to me. You think I don't have anything else to do right now? I'm in the middle of a move here, Michael. My stuff has been sent to Chicago and what am I doing? Making cocoa and clipping articles from *Architectural Review*? I don't have — You know, you amaze me. You're nothing but a — Yeah, I know you have kids.

And that's the point, wouldn't you want them to come and help you someday? Oh, man. You say that now. Yeah yeah yeah. You say that now. You know what? You know what you are? You're nothing but a spoiled rotten selfish little creep. You know that? That's all you are. You're just the worst person on the face of the earth. Forget it. That's all I have to — Forget it. This conversation is over. *(She hangs up)* Pathetic bastard. Rotten little son of a —

Joe enters.

JOE: You're here.

MELODY: Yeah.

JOE: What a lovely surprise.

MELODY: Is it?

JOE: Yes.

MELODY: Good. That's good.

JOE: Yes.

MELODY: Everything's good. Isn't it, Dad?

JOE: Yes. It's good.

MELODY: Yeah. Isn't it just a banner day ...

Slight pause.

JOE: You've been away, haven't you?

MELODY: Yeah, I've been away. You know that. I've told you twelve times now.

JOE: Of course. Tell me ...

MELODY: What?

JOE: Were you gone long?

MELODY: Oh, for crying — Yeah. I was gone three years.

JOE: Really?

MELODY:	Closer to four.
JOE:	Was it really?
MELODY:	Yes.
JOE:	To think!
MELODY:	Yeah ...

Slight pause.

JOE:	Where were you again? Was it the camp?
MELODY:	Camp?
JOE:	You know, the camp. What was the name of it again?
MELODY:	What camp?
JOE:	The camp. The church camp. The Anglican church camp ...
MELODY:	Harding?
JOE:	That's it. Exactly. Harding! Camp Harding. In the hills ... the what what what was the name of the hills again, the Cypress Hills?
MELODY:	The Cypress Hills.
JOE:	Exactly. The Cypress Hills. A beautiful spot. There was that lovely camp there. We sent you that one time. What was it — ?
MELODY:	Harding.
JOE:	Yes.
MELODY:	Camp Harding.
JOE:	Yes, of course. A beautiful spot.
MELODY:	I wasn't at Camp Harding, Dad.
JOE:	Were you not?
MELODY:	No. I was somewhere else. I was in Vancouver.
JOE:	Oh?
MELODY:	Yes.
JOE:	But not in ...

MELODY:	I was married, Dad.
JOE:	Married?
MELODY:	Yes. You remember. You gave me away.
JOE:	You got married at camp?
MELODY:	No. Not at camp. Since then.
JOE:	I see ... what was the name? I seem to have forgotten —
MELODY:	Camp Harding!
JOE:	No, not the camp. The boy.
MELODY:	The boy I married?
JOE:	Yes.
MELODY:	Charles.
JOE:	Charles?
MELODY:	You called him Charlie.
JOE:	Did I? Charlie ... that's right. Of course ... Charlie boy. Good old Charlie. With the funny eyes ...
MELODY:	But we broke up.
JOE:	Did you?
MELODY:	I told you.
JOE:	Things just don't last the way they used to ...
MELODY:	That's why I came here, dad. One of the reasons. Because we broke up. Because he tired me out. Bored me to tears until I couldn't stand it anymore. I couldn't stand Vancouver anymore. I can't stand this country anymore. I'm leaving. Well, I think I'm leaving. I'm supposed to start a job. I'm supposed to be somewhere else. And here we are talking about church camp. My God. You know Dad, I don't know what to do here. Like, maybe I need your support. Maybe I need to lean on you for a change ...
JOE:	There, there ...

MELODY: I know that the details slip away, but you
          could at least remember the big
          stuff. The life stuff. That wouldn't be asking
          too much .... Would it?

          JOE takes her hand.

JOE: It's always hard, isn't it dear?
MELODY: Yeah ... Even if you're not ... you know ...
          there's always doubt, and uncertainty, and
          regret ... It's not easy ...

          She starts crying. JOE comforts her.

JOE: There there there ... I wouldn't worry, my dear.
          It'll be all right ... everything will be all right
          ... There there .... Don't worry about ... Charlie
          .... He'll find a warm place to stay. And people
          who will feed him. And after a couple of days,
          he'll realize that he's not really at home and
          he'll make his way back. How do they do
          that? Their sense of smell, I suppose. It's truly
          remarkable, how they manage to make their
          way back. Remember we saw that movie!
          What was — ?
MELODY: *The Incredible Journey?*
JOE: That was it! That was it ... *The Incredible
          Journey*. A fine movie. How they get those
          animals to ... you know ... to act ... like that.
          It's incredible .... Anyway, little one. Don't you
          worry about ... it. Don't you worry about ...
          Charlie .... He'll come back .... He always does.
          Blackout.

End of Scene

Scene Eleven

> *Later. JOE is holding a copy of*
> Architectural Reviews, *and speaking*
> *to the audience. MELODY is very*
> *slowly cutting articles from the pile of*
> *magazines, putting them into folders*
> *which spill out around her on the floor.*

JOE: "The will of an epoch translated into space." Spandrels and mullions and I beams, neurons and axons and synapses ... a modulation in space beneath the glass surface of the skin .... One searches for a rhythmic regularity to one's work, one's life. All lightness and transparency, the Gothic and the classical fused into one, like the right brain and the left brain, creating the whole of the imagination, the will and the tension to hold these opposites, leading finally to serenity ... unsullied by memory ...

> *Lights shift slightly. JOE notices that*
> *MELODY is still there.*

JOE: I thought you were going ...
MELODY: I am.
JOE: When?
MELODY: Soon.
JOE: I've heard that before.
MELODY: Oh yeah ...
JOE: So when?
MELODY: When I'm ready to go. I know you made me promise I would leave — if you can even remember that. And I will leave — but only

	when I feel good about it. And I wouldn't feel good about it right now. It'll wait a few days ... And in the meanwhile ...
JOE:	Yes?
MELODY:	*(Indicating the magazines)* We have a lot to do.
JOE:	Yes.
MELODY:	So, I'll just stay for a while longer, OK?
JOE:	OK.
MELODY:	I'm not getting on your nerves or anything?
JOE:	No.
MELODY:	That's good.
JOE:	Am I? Am I getting on yours?
MELODY:	No.
JOE:	So you're OK.
MELODY:	Yeah. Are you?
JOE:	Yeah. I'm OK.
MELODY:	That's good.
JOE:	Yeah ... it's good ...
MELODY:	Help me with these ...

He sits down on the floor beside her, and together they start the long process of clipping and filing the relevant articles from many years of Architectural Review. *Slow fade to blackout.*

END OF PLAY

A CONVERSATION ABOUT THEATRE, DEMENTIA, AND TRANSFORMATION

With Sherry Dupuis, Pia Kontos, Julia Gray, and Christine Jonas-Simpson

—๛—

We are members of Collective Disruption, founded with the intention to disrupt dominant and oppressive cultural and social norms and imagine new possibilities for dementia care through the arts. Collective Disruption is a collaboration that brings together interdisciplinary researchers interested in aging and dementia, with a range of accomplished performing artists. *Sherry Dupuis* has a background in music and theatre but turned to participatory and social justice arts research to work for culture change in dementia care. *Pia Kontos* is a social scientist and health researcher who combines critical theory with performance and participatory arts to create a more just society for people living with dementia. *Christine Jonas-Simpson* is a nurse researcher who uses music, drama, painting, and documentary film to explore, share and understand how human beings transform through loss. *Julia Gray* is a playwright and director who has worked in professional theatre for many years and specializes in creating research-informed theatre for social change. One of the main outcomes of our Collective has been

61

Cracked: New Light on Dementia (Gray et al., 2017), a theatre project developed with the specific goal to challenge how we come to understand dementia as being irrevocably tragic. When we were approached by Eugene Stickland to contribute a piece to his book *No Harm Done,* we thought this would be an opportunity for us to share our reflections, experiences and insights working as a Collective. Here we offer a conversation about theatre and transformation in the context of dementia care.

Sherry: Using theatre as a means to explore and represent illness experiences is still pretty new in the Academy and Health Sciences. What drew each of us to theatre as a medium to explore dementia?

Christine: When Gail Mitchell, another member of Collective Disruption, and I saw, in a hospital auditorium, a research-based play about living with breast cancer, we were struck by the power of the medium. Engaging with the play was a visceral and emotional experience. It helped me question what I could do and stop doing to make a difference to the people I knew living with breast cancer. We saw the potential for our research about lived experiences of dementia to reach more people through theatre and in a way that opened conversation and provoked questions that could lead to new understandings and new ways of being.

Pia: For my doctoral research I conducted an ethnographic study of a long-term care home and was interested in embodied self-expression. By attending to the body in everyday life, I was drawn into a social and cultural world of relationships that seemed rather mundane and unexceptional, except when juxtaposed with the dominant tragedy discourse of dementia. There I found friendships, humour, creativity, conflict, and so much more that powerfully challenged assumptions of existential loss with dementia. I began thinking about how I could help others to see the rich social life that I had encountered with my research. I collaborated with a theatre director/playwright to create dramatized vignettes based on my research as a way to foster critical reflection amongst dementia practitioners about their assumptions and practices and about new possibilities for supporting people to live well with dementia.

Julia: It's a bit backwards for me because my home discipline is theatre. When I was doing my initial training, the emphasis was more on the professional arts for the sake of professional arts and the social message part of theatre depended on the theatre piece. That was something I was really interested in and so came to value and want to work in arts for social change.

Sherry: Directly following my music degree, I was hired to work in a long-term care home. I worked closely with people living with dementia and found I could connect with them through music in ways that others could not. I also witnessed conditions within the sector that made it challenging to provide compassionate care because of the focus on body care and tasks. It made me want to do something to change the culture. I went back to school, became a researcher, but discovered that there were structures within the Academy that were stifling my ability to support change. What is valued most in the Academy is published peer-reviewed articles and academic conference presentations, and I knew it would be difficult to shift the culture with only those types of outputs. Then, in 2002, I got a call from Christine and she said, "Gail and I are working on a play about dementia and we were wondering if you might want to join us." I jumped at the chance and from that day forward I found myself again because I was able to bring my passions for art, culture change, and research together.

Pia: When we all came together in 2011 on the *Cracked* project, the decision to use theatre was a pretty easy one and a necessary one given our collective commitment to challenging stigma and oppression. When you reached out to me about the idea of creating another play, I was really excited to explore how my research on the importance of the body for self-expression, interdependence, and reciprocal engagement might inform such a production because I saw it as an important way to challenge stigma.

Christine: The idea of relationality was really important to all of us, to use the play as a way to bring relationships to the forefront, recognizing what people living with dementia bring to those relationships and how relationships can shape experiences in profound ways and are key to supporting people to live well.

Julia: I remember one of the very first meetings we had as a team and this word 'relationships' kept coming up and I remember thinking, *What are they talking about?* Theatre is all about relationships so how is this play going to be any different from any other play because, of course, it was going to be about relationships. Through our discussions I came to understand that the current care culture isn't focused on relationships. We prize independence as opposed to interdependence. I got there eventually, but it was a weird moment for me personally.

Sherry: For me, relationality was important to explore in the context of dementia, but I wanted to look at relationality more broadly. As human beings in the world, we have relationships with so much more than just other human beings — with time, space, policies, institutions. I wanted the play to be able to capture the range of ways that relationality plays out in our lives that can provide opportunities or oppress. Did you see any similarities between the themes we wanted to explore in *Cracked* and themes in *Closer and Closer Apart?*

Julia: I thought there were really interesting parallels around how the medical culture was perceived and assumptions around that. There's the potential for medical culture to provide support, but that can often feel ostracizing and even oppressive; both plays touch on that. There is a wonderful monologue of Joe's where he's talking about how after they name what he has, they pretend they can fix 'it'. And that they take you away from what you know, and how you're a hero for taking a piss in the morning. That kind of infantilization happens within the medical culture and, because of that, he can't even use the word, what he feared he might be living with. It was the medical establishment that he feared the most. That's something we try to address as well. In *Cracked*, we see Elaine in many different ways. At first she is not sure who to share the diagnosis with, so she keeps it from everyone except her immediate family. But then she finds a community of other people living with dementia and is really thriving; she becomes an activist. It's the decision to move into institutional care where there is more fear than living with dementia itself, both for Elaine and her children.

Christine: The theme of complex relationships is clear in both plays. Frustration in relationship is portrayed so well by Melody in *Closer and Closer Apart* and Caroline in *Cracked* and we see sons who are either absent or so fearful that they can't help. The honest and complex realities of dementia shone through like we hear from people who see *Cracked*. Also, both plays show the new understandings that can come with dementia when raw authenticity emerges. For example, Melody learns of how proud her father Joe is of her after all these years when she did not think he had time for her. In *Cracked* we see that raw honesty in Clay and how hard it is for him to see his mom the way she is, but we also see how Carolyn grows through her experiences.

Pia: I too found that there was a lot of similarity between the two plays around the theme of relationships, particularly the ebbs and flows in relationships. For example, Melody is initially frustrated with Joe's struggles with his memory. I'm thinking of the scene where they are talking about Mrs. Hauser, and Melody says, "For God's sake Dad, you have to remember this." She seems to become more sympathetic when Joe says that he has to remind himself that Mom's dead and that he has trouble remembering her at all. She just goes with it rather than trying to correct him afterwards. His memory becomes less of a source of tension between them. Also, I thought it was interesting how they come to understand that they need each other. At the beginning Melody is focused on Joe needing her, but he says he'll be fine without her. He then expresses concerns about Chicago, which I think really was his way of expressing his desire for her to stay. Then there's also a shift with Melody, who admits to needing Joe but Joe pushes back by saying that Mrs. Hauser can handle the filing of the books and the periodicals, when they both know she won't be coming. Later he admits that maybe Melody could help him, and then she says maybe I need you too, and we see Joe comforting Melody. There is this constant movement with the shifting of the relationship between Melody and Joe, and ultimately what emerges is this mutual admission of the need and desire to be together.

Sherry: Another similarity that stood out for me is what Joe and Melody refer to as the 'family mythology', the idea that people living with dementia and their families have a past and create a shared history that is important to them as individuals and also to the construction of the family. I'm thinking about Elaine in *Cracked* and her history of lobster fishing with her brother and father and how that gets taken forward as an important aspect of her current life, and how Clay remembers his father and mother waltzing in the kitchen. That's part of their family history or 'family mythology' according to Joe and Melody. People with dementia have told me so often how, immediately following diagnosis, their histories, the fact that they might have cared for their own parents, and all the other roles they have had and expertise they have — that it's taken away, ignored the moment that a person is labelled with a dementia. They become just the dementia, just the 'patient'. You could see that history with Joe, his love of architecture and how important that is to his sense of self, and because of that, the close relationship he has with his periodicals and books. It is also an important part of his relationship with Melody.

Pia: One thing though that we haven't talked about yet is what the differences were between the two plays. Julia, you noted that there's a similar critique of the medicalization of dementia, particularly in how it fuels stigma and fear. But, I think that a critique of stigma and the ways that it legitimizes discriminatory policies and practices in the context of community-based care, including adult day programs and home care, and also residential long-term care is much more prominent in *Cracked*.

Sherry: Certainly the fear of naming 'it' that we see in *Cracked* is there for Joe, but we don't see as much of the absurd policies and the structural forces in the world that shape Elaine's and Vera's and their families' experiences and lives in significant ways. Given the importance of relationality to *Cracked*, we needed to use a relational, collaborative process ourselves. Let's turn to that.

Julia: What can be such a strength of any collaborative work is that you have the opportunity to draw and build on multiple perspectives. Obviously everybody and everything has limits, and to be able to really build an authentic trust with other people so that you can draw on each other's strengths and you can be pushed and challenged by others' experiences and perspectives will make a richer, hopefully, more full piece in the end. That requires humility to be able to really recognize our own limits. It also requires courage and the kind of trust where you can feel safe to really make mistakes and create things that maybe are not so polished. If you want to ultimately engage your audience in a deep way, then you need, as a collaborative team, to be able to work in that way and be deeply reflective. I think that speaks to theatre's strength — theatre by its very nature is a collaborative art form.

Sherry: What I loved about our process is the bringing together of such diverse individuals, social researchers, health researchers, and the professional actors and musicians who came in to do this collaborative work with us. I learned so much about myself through embodied enactment in movement and improv with the actors. Exploring themes from our research through music, facilitated by Tim Machin, our music director and one of the actors, provided us another opportunity to explore dementia in new ways. Those processes were critical to expanding my understanding of experiences of dementia in ways I know I would not have got to without this type of methodology.

Christine: I loved how we as researchers were welcomed by Julia and the actors to co-create scenes together. It was an organic process that was incredibly inspiring. I also loved our collaborations throughout the process with people living with dementia and their families to better understand what was most important to them. For example, when we created the placards with them in collaboration with visual artists as a means of telling the world what people living with dementia wanted the world to know about them, that was a powerful collective experience where emergence of new ideas and transformational moments were captured through art and conversation.

Pia: Like you, Sherry, I think the embodied engagement with the themes of the research and with our actual research data was such an important part of the process. I became much more emotionally connected to the material, as we were transforming it with movement, touch, speaking, and listening. It was a learning process to experience the meaning of the research through our senses; it's not something we do with traditional research methods. But this kind of collaboration is not easy, and I really do think the key to our success was Julia's extraordinary abilities as a theatre director. Julia worked so beautifully across the disciplines, facilitating communication between the artists and the researchers, and I think that was really key to the creation of the space of trust necessary to nurture our dialogue and foster critical reflection.

Christine: Staying true to the research findings while creating an aesthetically powerful piece can be extremely challenging.

Pia: With any interdisciplinary team there's going to

be different perspectives, and I think those differences bring a richness, but also bring challenges. With different perspectives, there's different interpretations and different priorities. As an example, Julia, you might recall there was a particular moment of tension that I think is worth us exploring here.

Julia: Yes, I remember Pia had brought in an article by cultural gerontologist Julia Twigg (Twigg & Buse, 2013) and there was some really evocative imagery in the article about the ways long-term care homes value easy means of clothing a person, such as putting people into Velcro. Ease of dressing and undressing is what was valued over individual preferences. We started to experiment with a series of rounds and generated some imagery to reflect some of the ideas in the article. We then shared our rough work with other team members who were not present when we had put it together, and some were really offended. Those of us who had generated the piece were taken aback by the response. I was certainly taken aback by it and not sure what to do with that emotion because I had assumed this was a place where we could explore, be kind of bad together, generate these things, and keep the best parts knowing most of it would get thrown out. So we all went away, slept on it, and when we came back I tried to reflect what I thought was happening, because none of us could articulate what was going on in that moment and why. We had a conversation about what made the scene offensive — there was confusion about whether we were critiquing this practice or reproducing the tragedy discourse by showing it in that way.

And, we agreed that we would work to be gentle with each other and that this was an important space to explore the darkness we know is also part of dementia and dementia care.

Pia: This seemed like a really important moment in our process. It was something we needed to experience in order to then be able to explore the absurdities of policy that were so important for us to expose and figure out how we could do it in a way we would all be comfortable with. We made the decision to make fun of them, show them for the absurdities they are. Upon reflection, it was an important process for us to work through, to figure out how we critique policies we think are harmful without reproducing the harm.

—∾—

This is also why theatre pieces are so important — they open up those broader conversations that prompt changes in actions.

—∾—

Sherry: I agree — conflict and tensions are often seen as problematic, but it is in those moments of tension and conflict that possibilities for seeing and acting anew can open up. Another moment of challenge that really stands out for me is when we first started to do public performances. We saw first-hand the emotional reactions people had, how they were moved in very deep ways. I remember the researchers saying, "Ethically we have to do something about this. We have to alert people in our introduction about how they might experience the play." We changed our introduction and when the actors heard the new introduction they were angry with us because they said, "That's what theatre is all about. It's supposed to move people and people will respond in different ways and all reactions should be welcomed." I thought the conversation we had after that happened was so important for everyone's understanding and helped us find a solution we all were comfortable with.

Pia: The play was doing exactly what we intended for it to do — to move audiences — but because our academic work doesn't typically move people in the way theatre does, it took some discussion for us to be comfortable with it.

Christine: And having that dialogue when those tensions did come up, opening a safe space for that to happen, was critical. For me it comes right back to the trust, and the relationships we had developed. Without that, we never would have had those conversations and learned from them. This is also why theatre pieces like *Closer and Closer Apart* and *Cracked: New Light on Dementia* are so important — they open up those broader conversations that then prompt changes in actions. When I hear university students change their words and images about persons living with dementia after seeing *Cracked*, it is incredibly hopeful. When students speak about how they will change and not be as afraid of people with dementia — including their own family members — it's a huge step on the culture change journey. I remember one time when we asked the audience what might change after seeing the play, a woman living with dementia put up her hand and said, "I will no longer hide." She said she had not told people other than her family that she had dementia. She added, "This is really a play about coming out." I love these unexpected gifts that shine hope.

Julia: To make change you need to move people. You need to have spaces where you can look at those assumptions and feel them, not just think about them but feel them and see them in different ways. Theatre, which has the potential to be so dynamic because it takes place in space and time, can do just that. Theatre can also reproduce harmful discourses. But it also holds the potential to bring forward voices often not heard, challenge harmful discourses, see oppression and stigma, and feel them in new and different ways.

Sherry: I remember after one of our early performances, an administrator of a long-term care home came up to us immediately following the performance and said, "That policy you showed in the play is in my home and I'm going back there now and I'm going to change it," and we all looked at each other and said, "That's what it's about," inspiring those changes.

Pia: It's also about activating the imagination. We can use this medium to critique, expose what's problematic, but the imagination is such an important part of this because we are working with audiences to envision new possibilities. Imagination is exactly what's needed to reimagine dementia.

Sherry: I think you're right, because people in dementia care settings are so embedded in the current culture that it is really hard for them envision the possibility that things could be different. But when they are able see things differently, see examples of what is possible, it can help them imagine possibilities for change. The scene in *Cracked* where Alex leans over and gently touches Elaine's hand to bring her back to washing the dishes is a good example. So many people have said, "It's just a simple touch that has so many possibilities."

Julia: Even for people to see their own stories played out in ways they haven't seen before, to see things they've experienced in their own lives, can be very validating and brings to the forefront things they want to share with other people but didn't feel they could.

Sherry: Or to see things never seen before. So many times when we perform *Cracked*, practitioners have said, "I've never seen the family before." That is shocking to us in one sense but in another sense it is understandable because they work in a very particular context where all the focus is on the person living with dementia; they don't see anything else. Then, we show a more complex, expanded picture, and dementia from different experiences and angles, like broadening the lens of a camera, and they can now see a fuller picture. They see the family and some of the experiences and inequities they face and begin to talk about the ways their practices are expanding to include the family. That is powerful stuff and why theatre is so important; when you see things differently, you act differently. So what are our hopes for culture change in dementia care?

Pia: My hope for the future is a society that actually

values relational caring, that makes human flourishing and relational capabilities the goal of caring and that resources are there to support this. I hope we can transform the unjust and harmful congregating, the separating, the confining of people living with dementia in care homes to alternatives that will support people to move freely in their communities, enjoy their rights to liberty, participate freely in the arts and in any other way that they desire to be engaged with social life. Ideally, I would love to see a shift from this control and isolation, punitive interventions, to inclusion, creativity, enjoyment and flourishing.

—❦—

The more we can embrace people living with
dementia, the more we can learn about life and
how to be present in the moment —
the only place where life is experienced.

—❦—

Julia: In relation to theatre making, I hope relationality can also be taken up there. There's often hesitation around relational practices in the theatre world, but it's a deep responsibility to tell people's stories and it has to be done relationally. Indigenous scholar Shawn Wilson (2008) writes beautifully about ideas of relational accountability. Storytelling is deeply relational, is a huge responsibility to be able to account for one's actions in those multiple ways.

Christine: Like Pia, my hope is for all care to be relational, compassionate and creative. Stigma continues to isolate people and families living with dementia. We keep asking, "How do we truly rid ourselves of stigma?" Theatre can help as we can see who we are and who others are and how we interrelate — we become the observer of ourselves and others — it provides space for us to reflect on how we see things, to question what we believe and how we might change our actions and ways of being. Also, the more we can embrace people living with dementia, the more we can learn about life and how to be present in the moment — the only place where life is experienced.

Sherry: For me, I long for a world and communities where all people living with dementia are seen as valued citizens in those communities and we see them for what they can bring to our lives. I hope that, through the relationships you all have talked about, we can create communities where people don't have to fear dementia because they know that the people around them will be there to help them navigate in the world, keep them safe, and support them in living life to the fullest. My other hope is that there can be many more collaborative processes such as ours, and, within the Academy, collaborative arts are seen as valued ways to generate new knowledge, expose social injustices in the world, and create a better world for everyone.

References

Dupuis, S.L., Kontos, P., Mitchell, G., Jonas-Simpson, C., & Gray, J. (2016). Re-claiming citizenship through the arts. Special Issue on Citizenship, Dementia: *The International Journal of Social Research and Practice,* 15(3):358-80.

Gray, J., Dupuis, S., Mitchell, M., Kontos, P., Jonas-Simpson, C., with Applewhaite, S., Kalamanski, L.N., MacLean, M., Muir, C., Prince, M., Machin, T., & Talbot, D. (2017). Cracked: new light on dementia. In J. Gray (Ed.), *ReView: an anthology of plays committed to social justice* (pp. 67-138). Rotterdam: Sense Publishers. https://crackedonde-mentia.ca/

Gray, J. Dupuis, S.L., Kontos, P., Jonas-Simpson, C., & Mitchell, G. (2020) *Knowledge as embodied, imaginative, foolish enactment: Exploring dementia experiences through theatre.* Forum Qualitative Sozialforschung / Forum: Qualitative Social Research, 21(3), Art. 2, http://dx.doi.org/10.17169/fqs-21.3.3444

Twigg, J., & Buse, C. (2013). *Dress, dementia and the embodiment of identity.* Dementia: The International Journal of Social Research and Practice, 12(3), 32-336.

Wilson, S. (2008). *Research is ceremony: Indigenous research methods.* Halifax & Winnipeg: Fernwood Publishing.

FADE TO LIGHT

A Play for a Darkened Venue

by

Eugene Stickland

INTRODUCTION TO
FADE TO LIGHT

—⁓—

I CAN'T REMEMBER how I met Dagmar Jamieson, exactly. I can't remember the where or when of it, but one day I just seemed to turn around and there she was and then it was like she had always been there.

Dagmar has Stargardt disease. Also called Stargardt macular degeneration, it is a genetic eye disorder which results in progressive loss of vision. She can see some, but not all. The centre of her vision is dark, she can only see through what we would think of as peripheral vision. (I will leave it to Drs. Bill Stell and Yves Sauvé and Dagmar herself to say more about it in their essay following the script.) I don't know that I ever found out much more about it than what I just wrote.

The condition didn't seem to be slowing Dagmar down any, from what I could tell. She was envisioning a gala event at the Hotel Arts. This was a major event, really. A gourmet meal with wine pairings — all the usual fixings, but just one catch: diners had to eat the meal blindfolded. Quite a trick, as it turned out. I was one of the diners that evening and it was one of the most unusual experiences of my life.

However, long before we ate that delicious meal in the dark, as it were, I was asked if I would write a play to be presented after that meal, the cornerstone of the evening, one could say. Well, if there was a way to say "No" to Dagmar, I hadn't found it, so I readily agreed. (And for the record, I did get paid for it, so my saintliness only runs so deep.)

I noticed looking through the program for the event that the play had been subtitled, *A Meditation on Vision*. I quite like that. None of the diners there that night wanted a technical lecture on macular degeneration, and if they had, I would have been the wrong person to ask. They wanted to be entertained.

My first question to Dagmar (well, I may have asked about the money first) was will they be wearing their blindfolds during the show. That decision was left to me, and I jumped at it — blindfolds on — for a number of reasons.

First, in terms of the production, it's a lot to expect of actors to memorize all those lines. It's not so bad and obviously part of the process if they have a run of a few weeks but for a one-off production, well I can't imagine you would find many performers willing to do that. With the audience blindfolded, I realize we could present it like a workshop production, with the actors sitting on stools, music stands for their scripts, with the piano player sitting just beside them.

Also, and maybe even more crucial given the fact that we didn't have a budget for such things, we wouldn't need sets, or costumes, or lights, or any of the many different things that you expect to see when you go to the theatre.

And finally, the magic! With the audience blind-folded, we could paint pictures and create scenes we never could have done on stage at a real theatre, let alone on a small, raised platform in a hotel banquet room. It took me back to plays I had written early in my career when there were such things — radio plays!

People may think radio plays are limited in scope, but in fact it's just the opposite. In a radio play you can go from *les rues de Paris* to the bottom of the deep blue sea to the rings of Saturn if you choose. You are only limited by your own imagination. And the wonderful thing is — and if you have ever listened to radio plays, often late at night when the house is quiet and you have only the comfort of the radio you will know this — the audience loves to go along on the journey.

In thinking about blindness — meditating on it, if you will — I must have had some insight (so to speak) into the nature of love and relationships. I must have been thinking about how hard it is to meet someone when you are harbouring some kind of disability. Let's face it, we all have our own kind of debilitating condition that others can't see when they look at us. There is always a moment of truth after we have met someone and can feel something fluttering inside our chest when we have to come clean and admit to our deficiency. And then we hold our breath: is this a deal-breaker, or will we move on?

Once I fully embraced the idea of a radio play, I let myself have some fun with the writing and make the narration story-book old-fashioned at times corny and over the top, but I believe it was entirely the right impulse. And I suppose in naming the characters simply

He and She, I was indicating that such a story could happen to any of us. After all, sooner or later, we all fall in love? Right?

A final thought. We recorded the three plays in this volume for an audio version of the book. The directing of the plays, which included casting, recording, trying to record in the middle of yet another lock down, choosing the music, etc. etc. etc. fell to an old friend of mine (in fact, I taught him when he was 14 years old), Aaron Coates. Among other activities too numerous to mention here, Aaron teaches acting classes for the Company of Rogues Actors' Studio in Calgary. (The

—⚬—

Creating an event with a
play at its centre
makes for a memorable evening.

—⚬—

same company figures in the production of *The Last Dance*, the final play in this collection.)

As Aaron was casting the plays, he met a young actress, Ashley King, who had lost her sight when she was twenty years old. She was trying to make her way in the theatre world, an arduous task for a full-sighted person, let alone for someone with any kind of disability. Aaron asked what I thought about casting her as SHE. I thought that it was incredibly important for us to cast her. If we are not doing such plays to foster awareness and promote understanding, then what are we doing?

Then we looked at it in light of this situation and I

wondered should I do a rewrite making the male character the sighted one so she could play the blind character. I wasn't sure how she would feel about that so we chatted on the phone and decided for a number of reasons to leave it as it is. And so we have a rather delicious irony in the casting of the recorded version — a blind performer in a play about blindness featuring a blind character which she doesn't actually play herself.

In the end, we are left with two human beings running across a big park in a rainstorm. One is blind. The other instinctively serves as his guide. This to me is the heart of the play. This to me is the hope for the human race: that we celebrate our similarities, and not dwell on our differences; that we recognize our strengths and not dwell on our perceived weaknesses.

FADE TO LIGHT

Fade to Light was commissioned by Dagmar Jamieson and the In/Sight Dining in the Dark committee in aid of the Foundation Fighting Blindness.

It was performed on October 2, 2008 at Hotel Arts in Calgary, Alberta with the following cast and personnel:

Narrator .... Grant Reddick
He .... Tony Binns
She .... Jennifer Roberts
Pianist..................................... Gloria Kae Macrae

Director................................... Eugene Stickland
Producer .... Janet St. Germain
Sound .... Luke Moar
Original Score .... Gloria Kae Macrae
(with two selections by Ira Gershwin)

Fade to Light

Fade to Light is meant to be experienced in total darkness. It was commissioned by Dagmar Jamieson for the IN/Sight: Dining in the Dark fundraiser in Calgary, Alberta

Characters

The Narrator
He
She

A Piano, played

Also, some sound effects, especially of the thunderstorm that meanders in and out of the story.

NARRATOR: Lights fade to black.
And although the light has faded, our vision has not.
If we are able to see with our mind's eye,
We will see a large urban park, verdant
Under a delicate robin's egg fragile prairie sky.
Oh, we might also see a few storm clouds on the horizon
And even cue the thunder—

Slight pause. No thunder.

I say, we might even cue the thunder—

A dull rumble of thunder is heard.

Thank you. But the storm is still a long ways off,
Has barely entered into the collective consciousness
Of the people busy at work and at play in the park
Whom we now see for ourselves on the insides of our eyelids.

From far but not too far away,
We hear the playing of a piano, softly,
    Melodic and gentle—

Slight pause. Nothing.

I say, from far and away,
We hear the playing of a piano

> *The piano can be heard to play, and
> continues to play underneath, initially
> quite abstract and atmospheric.*

Thank you. And so with the piano playing
And the storm at bay for now, at last
We begin our story.

> *Under the next speech, the sounds he is
> describing become audible.*

Fade to black.
The sound of a piano.
The sound of perhaps birds.
And not to put too fine a point on it
The distant laughter of children
And the gentle rustling of leaves.

For it is summer.
And it is a park.
Where in there is a green bench.
Upon which She sits.
And into the near proximity of her on the
green bench
He can be seen to enter.

For this is a simple story of him and her
He and She.
If we could see Him

We would see that He has his suit jacket
Which is rather blue thrown over his shoulder
In the style and manner of people who do
such things;

While She if we could see
Wears a pale blue sun dress
Simple, yes, but lovely in its simplicity.

Yes, if you could see her for yourself
You would see that she appears to be
What they used to say rather quaintly and
naively,
Fetching.

And maybe it has to do with her fetchingness
Or maybe for that matter it doesn't
Because we could hardly say He is on the
make
But be that as it may
Instead of passing by
He lingers by her green bench
Thinking as if suddenly
That this just might be
The best place in all the world
To stop and sit and rest his weary feet
And everything else attached to his feet
Weary and otherwise.

And so He stops
And He seems to regard her

With such benevolence and innocence as He
can muster
In other words, not meaning to creep her,
For He is no creep, He
And so He stands there a moment
In the attitude of one regarding another
Yet She makes no attempt to look at him, at all
And so He clears his throat.

HE: A-hem.
NARRATOR: And then She looks up at him
And He smiles
Although She doesn't smile
Although She doesn't not smile, either
Causing him to scratch his head
As men will do when interpreting mixed
signals
In particular those emanating from the fairer
sex
And yet He decides to muster up his courage
For once in his life and
Seize the day
And go for it
And so He says:
HE: Excuse me. I was wondering if you'd mind
sharing your bench with me, just for a little bit
NARRATOR: To which She says:
SHE: It's not my bench, actually.
HE: Oh?
SHE: I believe it belongs to the city.
HE: I see.

NARRATOR: Although He was not really seeing much of
anything
And certainly had no way of knowing
If what she had said was a yes or an in fact no.

She only looked at him in a rather enigmatic
manner
And because He was still in the throes of *carpe
diem*
(And besides, his feet were sore
And his back was aching)
He sat down right there on the bench beside
Her
Throwing as they say, caution to the winds
Devil take the hind most and all the rest of it.

And so there they sat.

And He let out a long groaning sigh of relief
just for being off his feet.
HE: Ahhhhhhhh   hh-mmmmm-ghghghgh . . . . .
NARRATOR: And there they sat, so close
And yet so distant.
The Piano began to play
In perhaps a local café
Piano begins to play, perhaps something by
Gershwin.
Or at least someone began to play the piano
Because everyone knows pianos can't play
themselves
Although neither He nor She
Could see this

	They could only hear the perhaps Gershwin

They could only hear the perhaps Gershwin
And other tunes they could not quite put
Their individual finger or collective fingers
on.

HE: Nice music.

NARRATOR: Said He, to which She replied:

SHE: Yes, indeed.

> *Pause of several seconds as they listen to
> the piano player. We can also hear the
> ambient sounds of the park.*

NARRATOR: And even as we look inward
Peering into the darkness
Still we perhaps perceive the dappled light
Filtered through the leaves of stately trees
Standing sentinel around and behind the
little green bench
The light illuminating the blue clothing of the
one
And the blue clothing of the other
And we catch perhaps out of the corner of
our eye
The darting of a bird
Or the flickering frayed flight of a butterfly
And above all that
Pillowy white clouds floating on high
Across the blue dish of the sky.

And while the piano player played
And the leaves trembled
And the clouds floated by on high

A deafening silence surrounded
The Man and the Woman on their little green
bench
For while he had summoned up the courage
To sit down in the first place
He now found himself falling victim
To a certain unwelcome silent affliction
That had plagued him all of his adult life
For which he compensated
By working too hard, making in the process
Astronomical sums of money from which
He derived surprisingly little satisfaction.

And now here it was again.
His tongue was tied, his mind was locked up
tight.
And try as He might, He had no thought
Of anything to say
Nothing coherent anyway.

For her part, She just sat there
Staring straight ahead—
What was she looking at, anyway?
It was hard to tell. What was She thinking,
anyway?
Impossible to tell.
She may have been trying to recall
The capital of Arkansas
Or the middle name of a former lover
For all He could tell.
In point of fact, at that very moment

That He was wondering what She was
wondering.
She was wondering why a man such as He
Would have the temerity to join her thusly
Yet not follow up with some kind of
conversation
No matter how banal, mundane, trivial.

And this would hardly be the first time
In the entire history of relationships
Between men and women that the woman,
To compensate for the inadequacies of the
man,
Would take the as it were bull by the horns
And get the as it were ball rolling by saying:

SHE: Isn't it a lovely view from here?
NARRATOR: And after a brief pause
              During which there was almost an audible
              clunk
              As his brain clicked into gear
              He replied, ever so eloquently:
HE: Yep.
NARRATOR: She waited for more
              But more was not forthcoming.
              And so there they sat in silence
              Filled only by the indefatigable piano player
              But even she seemed to fall victim
              To this malaise
              For her playing became softer

              It does.

And slower.

It does.

And she even faltered and hit a few wrong
notes.

She does.

And then she just gave up entirely
And for a while there was no more music.
And all was still, until there was heard in the
distance

We hear the rumble of thunder.

The faint rumble of thunder.
And then She may have forgotten herself
for a moment
And the awkwardness of the situation
And maybe it was because she could sense
No bad energy or strange vibrations
Originating from the man beside her—
In fact it suddenly felt to her
That they had always known each other
There was just something so familiar about
him,
And so She said:

SHE:	Sounds like that piano player got spooked by the thunder.
NARRATOR:	To which He said:
HE:	Actually, the music stopped before the thunder.
SHE:	Maybe the lightning then.

HE:	Maybe.
SHE:	You can see the lightning before you hear the thunder because light travels faster than sound.
	But I suspect you already know that.
HE:	I may have heard that before, all right.
NARRATOR:	And then She said:
SHE:	Well, I hope he plays some more.
NARRATOR:	To which He said:
HE:	She.
SHE:	She?
HE:	The piano player.
SHE:	The piano player is a "she?"
HE:	Yes.
SHE:	How can you tell? We can't see him from here.
HE:	Can't see her.
SHE:	Whatever.
HE:	The piano player is a she. Don't ask me how I know. I just do.
NARRATOR:	And at that exact moment, the piano player
	Who was in fact a she
	Began playing again
	Seemingly, soundingly recovered from what had
	Thrown her off the keys in the first place
	To which She of the park bench said:
SHE:	Well, would you look at that. Speak of the devil. There he is again.
NARRATOR:	To which He said:
HE:	She.
NARRATOR:	And then there was another clap of thunder, closer

	To which she said:
SHE:	I hope it doesn't rain.
HE:	Why?
SHE:	Because we'd get wet.
NARRATOR:	To which He said nothing, and so there they sat,
	Dry, at least, listening to the almost familiar song on the piano
	With the thunder storm rolling across the open expanse
	Of park and river valley that spread out before them
	Illuminated in a perfect shaft of Hallmark sunlight
	Fanning through the billowy, ever more leadening clouds.
	There were buildings beyond the reaches of the park
	And at length She remarked on them, saying:
SHE:	I like when you can see the foliage of the trees against the buildings like that, like over there, to the right.
NARRATOR:	She indicated "over there, to the right"
	With a subtle movement of her right shoulder
	Which He either saw or didn't see
	On any account, He didn't look but He did say:
HE:	It's the best of both worlds, nature and architecture. I think I see what you mean. I don't really like nature, like the uncut thing, camping and all that nonsense, sleeping with a tree root digging into your kidneys, the bugs

and all the rest of it. But at the same time, I find the city gets to be too much at times, the traffic, all the noise, especially the sound of trucks and motorcycles and inane conversations you can't help overhear in cafes and one-sided cell phone conversation where all they ever say is "where are you, where are you, where are you?" Yeah, well, so anyway, to have the best of both worlds like that, the trees and the buildings, that seems like a good thing ...

NARRATOR: To which She said:

SHE: It's a question of balance.

NARRATOR: To which He said:

HE: Exactly.

NARRATOR: And so they sat some more feeling quite satisfied

With themselves both individually and collectively

And with seemingly renewed enthusiasm

The piano player launched into a new song

That seemed to capture the moment to the point

That if this, their spontaneous blind date—

And we employ the expression cautiously—

Were to come to anything and lead

To subsequent encounters in the days

And weeks and months and years to come

And they were to look back over the vista of time

At this precise moment, they would remember

Every note and nuance of the song and together

Hereinafter think of it as "their song."

	And then He said to her:
HE:	So other than the buildings rising up beyond the foliage of the trees, what else do you see?
SHE:	You mean, what do I spy, with my little eye?
HE:	Something like that.
NARRATOR:	To which She said:
SHE:	I spy with my little eye, something that is ... orange.
HE:	OK. So what is it?
SHE:	You have to guess.
HE:	I see.
SHE:	Go ahead.
HE:	Look. I have to warn you. I'm not very good at this game.
SHE:	It's just a kids' game.
HE:	Not to me, it's not.
SHE:	Look, I made it easy for you. It's not like there's a lot of orange stuff out there. Go ahead!
HE:	OK. Uhh. Is it the sun?
SHE:	No, it's not the sun. You can't use the sun in a game of I spy. A person would fry their eyes out. Anyway, other than in a kid's painting, the sun is hardly orange. It's more of a yellow. Not that anyone really knows for certain given that you can't actually look at it. It's like looking at the face of God which you can't do and everyone knows if you even try to look at the face of God He will turn you into a pillar of salt. Which can't be good for your skin. Do you believe in God?
HE:	I think so. Maybe. Kinda. I'm not sure. Do you?

SHE:	I'm spiritual without being religious.
HE:	You hear that a lot these days.
SHE:	Yeah. I put it on my profile of a dating site I belong to. Plenty of Fish, they call it.
HE:	Any luck?
SHE:	Not yet. It's been catch and release so far ...
HE:	I see ...
NARRATOR:	The wind blew gently over the couple on the bench
	Cooling and calming as they sat listening
	To the person playing the piano:
SHE:	It's a He.
HE:	No way: She.
NARRATOR:	The notes drifting across the open expanse
	And then at length, She said:
SHE:	It's the Frisbee.
HE:	What is?
SHE:	The orange something which I spied with my little eye is the orange Frisbee those two guys are throwing. And never catching.
HE:	Ahhhh . . . I see.
SHE:	You see it?
HE:	I see what you're talking about.
SHE:	OK. Your turn.
HE:	For what?
SHE:	I spy.
HE:	Oh.
SHE:	Go ahead.
HE:	I don't know.
SHE:	Go ahead. Before it rains.
HE:	I already told you, I'm not very good at it.
SHE:	There's nothing to it.

HE: Actually, there is.
SHE: What?
HE: Spying.
SHE: What are you talking about?
HE: Seeing.
SHE: Yeah?
HE: Yeah.
SHE: What about it?
HE: I have a condition.
SHE: Oh?
HE: A situation.
SHE: Oh.
HE: Yeah.
SHE: I see.
HE: Yeah.
SHE: OK ...
NARRATOR: They sat in silence for a moment
            as She processed this information.
            Was He putting her on?
            She'd seen him walk up to the bench
            With her own two eyes.
            He was hardly a stumbling bumbling
            Shuffling forlorn figure
            Creeping through the great dark void
            Of the earth, a white cane at the advance.

            He was a vital, vibrant even handsome young
            man
            Seen in the right light, but surely
            That can be said for all of us.

If She could manage to reel something like
him in
On Plenty of Fish, she'd do it in a heartbeat
And perhaps have him and hold him for the
long haul
Depending on his taste in music
And of course his personal hygiene habits.

Meanwhile, the storm had meandered out
To the edge of town and then had a change of
heart
And was now headed back toward them
With renewed vigour and enthusiasm,
Announcing its return with an impressive
Flash of cracked light and a sudden clap of
thunder.

We hear the thunder, louder than before.

In response to the lightning and thunder She
said:

SHE:	That storm's coming back around.
NARRATOR:	To which He said:
HE:	So I hear.
NARRATOR:	The wind began to pick up a little

Rustling and ruffling leaves
And easily swaying the long branches of trees
And if one had a nose for such things
One could detect the trace of perhaps rain on
the air.

For her part, She wanted to learn more about

	His mysterious situation or condition
	But being a mannered young woman
	She couldn't find the words to ask him,
	Couldn't imagine the words with which to ask.
	For his part
	He couldn't help but think:
HE:	Oh boy. OK. Here we go. Here we go again. Here it comes. Here comes the deal-breaker, if ever there was one. How was I to know?
NARRATOR:	How was he to know there would be someone here
	Sitting on his bench?
HE:	Every day I come here.
NARRATOR:	Everyday He comes here.
	Everyday He sits here alone
	Happy to do so.
HE:	Quite happy to do so, thank you very much.
NARRATOR:	And now this.
HE:	And now this ...
NARRATOR:	Now he could feel himself being drawn into
	The cold grey maze of the same old story
	He'd told a million times before
	Not even a story He had chosen for himself
	But one that had chosen him, after all.

Just as he started to speak, another crack of thunder.

Another crack of thunder.

To which She said:

SHE:	Now that's getting quite close.

HE: Yes, it is.
SHE: We're quite vulnerable up here.
HE: Yes, we certainly are.
NARRATOR: The clouds closed over above them
           And the wind picked up its pace
           And they suddenly seemed all alone in the
           world
           Together, together yet alone,
           Like a couple traveling together in a foreign
           land
           And isn't it funny and wonderful at the same
           time
           Just how quickly and completely that can
           happen
           When the planets align and circumstances
           conspire
           To create the perfect conditions for that
           phenomenon
           We call love at first sight?

           She felt it.
           He felt it.

           In fact, such a feeling could only be felt by one
           If it was being felt by the other, a closed circuit
           The current flowing back and forth, each to
           each.

               Thunder is heard, quite loud. Wind in the
               branches, rustling leaves.

           And yet for all that,
           The electric current and the unspoken bond,

They each knew they had some unspoken
business
To attend to, in particular the young man
Who had left his business unspoken in the
first place
And now had no alternative but to find the
Articulation for it, and as they say, come
clean.

HE: Well, here we go ...

SHE: Sorry?

HE: Look, I'm sorry I couldn't play along with you
earlier, you know, I spy and all that.

SHE: It's OK. It's such a silly game, anyway.

HE: Well, to me it seems like the coolest game
ever. It's not the game, you see, it's me ...

NARRATOR: He trailed off and felt the first perhaps drop
of rain fall
On the back of his right hand
And He heard the roar of thunder from on
high
Urging him to get on with it
Before the heavens opened up
And a hard rain fell upon them.

To put it in Shakespearean terms
Even as He felt that drop on rain on his right
hand
Which at the moment was busy
Wringing the fingers of his left hand
He screwed his courage to the sticking place
And charged on ahead
While for her part

She waited patiently for him to do so
Hoping He would screw his courage and
charge on ahead
Before the rains came and the wind blew her
hair
Into something resembling a robin's nest—
She having just hours before visited her stylist
And was looking quite good if she did say so
herself
Although her companion hadn't said anything
Which was typical on many levels
And then another peal of thunder was heard,
closer,
Following on the heels of, if it could be seen,
A sharp flashing of lightning ripping its way
Through a deeply leadened violet cloud.
And then He said:

HE: As a child I could see, but then a darkness
began to appear at the centre of things pushing
my perception to the periphery. We went to
the doctor and we learned that my parents had
within them a recessive gene that led to this,
like they had both   come to the picnic
but neither of them had thought   to bring
the sandwiches, at least as far as my vision is
concerned. But I remember the things I've
seen and I'm sure I've seen an orange Frisbee
against a backdrop of green, I'm sure that's in
the image bank, but I do not see it now.

SHE: But you walked to this bench. I saw you.

HE: Yes. 125 steps from the fountain. More or less.

SHE: I see. Oh. Sorry, I didn't mean that. I mean I
understand.

HE: That's OK. We all see in our own way.

NARRATOR: There was a profound truth to that

           Or so it seemed to her

           And She felt for all the world that

           Something had been shared between them

           Something subtle and unseen

           And yet something bright enough and clear enough

           To cause her to reach out and take his right hand

           In her own much smaller right hand

           And give it a little squeeze as if to say

           I am here.

SHE: I am here.

HE: Yes, I am aware of that.

SHE: Right. Sorry . . .

HE: There are men and women who know how to get down into the double helix of the DNA and fix this. You wouldn't believe the science. It's like science fiction. You can't believe the stuff they dream up. And the amazing thing is that they're actually getting somewhere. It's actually working. They restored the sight of a dog, and of a man, just in one eye in case it backfired, but he can now make out the outline of a leaf with that eye. And I just hope they figure it all out in time for it to do some good for me. But then again, it's been my experience that hope can be a very torturous thing.

SHE: You can't stop hoping.

HE: I hate to get my hopes up in case it all falls apart.

SHE: I won't let you stop.

HE:	You don't even know me.
SHE:	I feel like I do.
NARRATOR:	At that moment there was a tremendous flash of lightning
	And a great clap of thunder all at the same moment

We hear the thunder.

	And finally the rain began to come down in earnest.
	She renewed her grip on his hand and said:
SHE:	I can't let you go back the 125 steps to the fountain, there's no protection.
HE:	But that's the only way I know for sure.
SHE:	It's a lot closer to the restaurant. We can get a cup of tea or something and see for ourselves if that piano player's a man or a woman.
HE:	Ok. If you're sure.
SHE:	I'm sure. Let's go before we get soaked and my hair is ruined completely.
HE:	OK. Thanks.
SHE:	Let's go.
NARRATOR:	And so, if we would see, even with our eyes shut
	If we would see in our mind's eye
	Each in our own way
	A young couple, So close to being all alone in the world
	And yet so close to being perhaps alone no more
	Running, hand in hand,
	Haltingly, yet hurriedly traversing

A great lawn in an urban park
Against a backdrop of swaying and rustling
trees.
A wind impeding their progress
And the rain lashing against them.

A rather rustic restaurant, soft lights gleaming
Into burled wood awaiting them,
All the while, their brief journey underscored
By the sounds of the piano.

We hear the rain storm, more thunder, and
the piano for about twenty seconds as we
follow their progress in our mind's eye.

And does it matter, after all, they're just one
Small and insignificant not even couple
swimming
In the great sea of humanity; does it matter
That He can't see or that She cares enough
About the fortunes of a stranger
To guide him across the great unknown
expanse of lawn?

It is after all the great blessing of humanity
That hope will lie like a seed dormant
And unseen even in the most generous of
hearts
And yet, we must believe, it never dies
Rather it thrives and so causes us to open our
eyes
And as our vision fades into light

Let us never stop seeing that there is
Hope and mercy in the world, always, still.

The piano concludes as the storm fades.

NARRATOR: And so we fade to light.
End of play.

And we fade to light.

END OF PLAY

—⚉—

REFLECTIONS ON
FADE TO LIGHT

With William Stell, Dagmar Jamieson,
and Yves Sauvé

—∿—

DR. WILLIAM STELL

"A DARKNESS began to appear at the centre of things," but "there are men and women who know how to fix this." Yes!

As a vision scientist for nearly sixty years, I've spent most of my time trying to understand how we perceive light — how the retina senses and decodes images of scenery, implements, faces, electronic devices, and so on. As a young faculty member in the Jules Stein Eye Institute (UCLA) during the 1970s, I was surrounded by researchers and eye docs whose main goal was to understand, prevent, and cure inherited retinal degenerative diseases such as retinitis pigmentosa (RP) and Stargardt's disease. For the most part, though, I focused on basic discovery rather than clinical treatments and cures.

After moving to Calgary, Alberta in 1980, I became more interested in learning and doing something about inherited retinal disease. Several factors conspired to make this happen. I came as Director of the Lions Sight Centre (University of Calgary Faculty of Medicine) — supported by huge fundraising efforts of the Lions Clubs of District 37, and staffed by Drs. Art Spira, Rick Hanna, Pat Wyse, and Peter Price.

Their enthusiasm and commitment inspired me more than I can say. Through this I met a group of bikers who gave their time to raising money for sight research through an annual motorcycle Ride For Sight, in which I partici- pated — no, not as a rider, but as a volunteer helping with the event. The Ride, in turn, was, and still is, the signature fund-raising event for the Retinitis Pigmentosa Research Foundation, now called Fighting Blindness Canada, a charity based in Toronto whose mission was to support research on RP.

In 1989, the Foundation made a commitment to sup- porting the best of relevant research and research training in Canada by instituting a stringent, competitive program of peer-reviewed research. I was invited to become the first Chair of the Scientific Advisory Board, to oversee the review of research grant proposals by a panel of experts in the field, and did so for six years. Later on I served several more years with the Foundation as Director of Research Programs, and then Expert Scientific Advisor for almost ten years. Finally, in the past twenty years I joined a facul- ty colleague, Dr. Torben Bech-Hansen, in research on his animal model of Congenital Stationary Night Blindness.

This wonderful network of experiences with RP pa- tients, researchers, and fundraisers is what got me involved with the two experts who join me in this chapter. First you will meet someone who has Stargardt's disease, who has learned to live with it since she was a teenager, and who was the instigator of the Foundation's fundraising event, "Insight: Dining In The Dark," which led Eugene Stickland to write the play, *Fade To Light*: Dagmar Venclik Jamieson.

DAGMAR JAMIESON

I REMEMBER MYSELF as a young, skinny twelve-year-old sitting in the back of the classroom at St. Mary's elementary school, so happy to reconnect with my friends whom I'd missed seeing all summer. I enjoyed sitting at the back of the class with my friends; I felt cool that I fit in. Yet, this was the year I became aware that something wasn't quite right. I was unsure why the teacher's face was somewhat blurry and the words on the blackboard were hard to read.

Was there something wrong with my sight? I hadn't noticed anything wrong with my sight during the summer holidays — at least, nothing as prominent as at my first day back at school. Was it nerves?

My expectations in grade six were normal for my age. I was a stick-like girl hoping to fit in with the cool girls and expecting to flirt with the boys. I was not as voluptuous as the popular girls. Striving to be popular in grade school was unfamiliar to me.

Weeks later, sitting in the ophthalmic chair, hearing the doctor voice the words, "You are losing your sight" was alarming to say the least.

The first time I had ever faced a challenge as frightening as this was when I moved with my family from Czechoslovakia to Austria at the age of eight. There I was expected to integrate into a classroom in which I didn't speak the same language. With a creative imagination, I strived to find solutions to problems. I tried hard to speak the language, but couldn't figure out how to reorganize the letters to sound like German, as I did with pig Latin (a common game I played with my friends, trying to develop secret words). In time I learned how to speak German, but I expected a lot of myself through this adaptation of fitting in with the rest of the students who spoke and understood the language. When report cards were distributed by the teacher, Frau Stirn, tears filled my eyes, staining my cheeks. I was afraid that I wasn't going to pass the grade, and what would I say to my parents? Life was difficult enough. I'd lost my friends, relatives, and most of all my grandma when I left my homeland, Czechoslovakia. I felt scared and alone dealing with these challenges.

Not only that, but eight months later my parents started to speak about moving yet again. I was beginning to grasp the language, and my grades reflected the success I was achieving. I felt like I was beginning to fit in. Suddenly I was in Canada starting from scratch, learning to speak a foreign language again. Fellow students laughed at me for mispronouncing "potatoes" as "bodado," which sounded the same to me.

By the time we reached Canada, I was legally blind, only able to see the letter E at the top of the eye chart. Sitting in the doctor's chair, I imagined myself navigating the world while being blind. I insisted on overcoming this situation by adapting, just as I did learning to speak first German and then English. I did it then, so why could I not learn to adapt to not seeing?

I proceeded to ride my bicycle, ski black diamond runs, figure-skate dance, and many other activities that other teenagers engaged in. Most people didn't notice that I was blind. This started to become my secret. Of course, some thought there was something awkward about me, especially when I didn't recognize others waving at me or trying to engage with me. Being a teenager, I preferred to be identified by others as simply different, rather than blind. A mature person may think that is a silly compromise. However, I just wanted to be like everyone else.

Eventually, I realized that being different meant being unique, which I reframed into a good thing. By adjusting to new ways of being, I developed new neural pathways which enhanced my entrepreneurial thinking. I explored being a proprietor in various ventures. As an out-of-the-box thinker, I deliberated with many creative ideas.

"You are blind," some would say; but I am a visionary, and sight is not necessary! As a visionary who cannot see, I learned that I could see with my imagination. I simply enhanced my imagination in order to cope with being blind.

At the age of 45, I met Dr. Ian MacDonald, who inspired me with the hope in research that is striving to cure blindness. This opened my mind to future possibilities. I am a dreamer. No matter how long it can take to bring my dreams to fruition, I believe anything is possible. I am always hopeful, because when you put your imagination into action, the possibilities are endless.

I wanted to be part of the quest to find a cure to end all blindness, so I asked Dr. MacDonald to connect me with the Foundation Fighting Blindness (FFB). They proceeded to inform and educate me about the various inherited forms of blindness. I wanted to help, so I did, by organizing various fundraising events to raise awareness regarding the ongoing research as well as to raise funding in support of these research ventures. Research takes time and money, but the hope is definitely evident. I know somehow, in some way, blindness will be curable. There is much promise in research developments such as gene therapies, as well as many other promising discoveries.

In many ways, technology has afforded me, in many ways, to function without sight. I use the GPS so as not to get lost navigating cities I am unfamiliar with. Speech-to-text aids my ability to write. Key echo is another tool that allows me to hear what I am typing. Voice-over features on computers read text within many computer applications.

My world is now open to knowledge, communication, and connection. This is the miracle I dreamed about many years ago, before text-to-speech was a common function. Autonomous vehicles are also becoming a possibility to amplify my independence.

The FFB introduced me to Dr. William Stell, who sat on the advisory board for research. Dr. Stell then introduced me to Dr. Yves Sauvé, as well as many other brilliant researchers. It is exciting and very empowering to meet these exceptional individuals. I am a bold dreamer, and I never underrate the possibilities of dreams. With this lavish imagination my dreams are audacious, as in my favourite quote by Albert Einstein: "Imagination is more important than knowledge. For knowledge is limited, whereas imagination embraces the entire world, stimulating progress, giving birth to evolution." I believe anything is possible; one just needs to focus one's mind on the possibility.

These days, as a blind individual, I become frustrated with mundane issues. In crowded social settings it can be difficult to connect with others, which can make me feel alone and disconnected. Don't get me wrong, I am a very social person, not shy to step up and start a conversation with anyone. But I can feel awkward when in a situation where I am not able to discern the interest to engage in conversation. These quirks affect many individuals in various ways. I underestimate how many people feel the oddities, not just because of lack of vision, but perhaps due to other limiting afflictions.

"Insight: Dining in the Dark," one of the fundraising efforts that I orchestrated with a great team of volunteers, was a very enlightening experience. We commissioned Eugene Stickland to write a play for the evening and he gave us *Fade to Light*, a poignant play which showcases some of these awkward moments. One of the most relevant observations I connected with was not being able to communicate visually with others. Imagine not being able to assess a situation but needing to be brave enough to dive right in without that sufficient information.

In the play, when the character "He" sat down on the bench beside the lady, he imagined having a conversation — not knowing if she was even interested in having one with him. He courageously reveals his differences in a non-self-sabotaging way. I felt that playwright Eugene was brilliant in portraying these moments of struggle.

To my surprise, the "Insight: Dining in the Dark" evening brought to light many such moments. After the event, many of my friends who attended the evening reflected upon their experience and the challenges they noticed while being blindfolded — being able to interact in a conversation blindfolded at a round table, not aware of who is listening or looking at you while you attempt to engage in a conversation with them. Perhaps the flavours of the food and drink were more intense, and this became a pleasant surprise. Certain aspects of not having visual clues are quite refreshing.

Fade to Light is a poetic reflection of the awkward moments one has to face when one is a square peg in a round world. I believe most of us are unique; however, I will admit personally I have struggled to fit in throughout most of my life, regardless of my differences.

Back to William Stell

SPEAKING OF "INSIGHT," let me thank you, Dagmar, not only for sharing this enlightening account of your experience having Stargardt's disease, but also for your insight into how it effects you — you as an intelligent, energetic and optimistic 'do-er', facing the restrictions to your activities and outlook with courage and hope.

Next we will learn more about that disease and the research that's bringing hope to sufferers of RP, Stargardt's, and other inherited retinal degenerative disorders. Let me introduce Dr. Yves Sauvé, who was mentioned by Dagmar and who has personal experience doing the kind of research supported by Fighting Blindness Canada.

Dr. Sauvé, please tell us about your experience as a researcher. What is the biological problem or defect in Stargardt's disease? What are we learning about it from laboratory research? And what are the prospects of restoring at least some vision to those who have lost it to retinal disease?

DR. YVES SAUVÉ

PICTURE THIS: on July 1, 2005, my family and I are driving from Salt Lake City to Edmonton. As we cross the border, we are welcomed by a hailstorm. Our return home to Canada will be marked forever in my mind: boundless challenges and opportunities await us. Having been headhunted from the Moran Eye Center to the Department of Ophthalmology at the University of Alberta by then-chair Dr. Ian MacDonald, I will be introduced to Stargardt.

My mission impossible, which I did accept before the message self-destructed, is to study the events that underlie the progressive loss of central vision in this blinding disease. Serendipitously, my Utah colleague Dr. Kang Zhang has just genetically engineered a mouse that mimics the disease. He generously allows me to bring along not three but eight blind mice to establish my own colony in Edmonton. Thanks to generous financial supports from the Canadian Institutes of Health Research and the Alberta Heritage Foundation, I get all the toys that will allow me to delve into this fascinating world: the retina. I am all set.

With the invaluable assistance of Ms. Sharee Kuny, we examine this thin layer that lines the back of the eye. In human and Stargardt mice, the cells responsible for colour vision (cone photoreceptors) become dysfunctional and die progressively with age. The big question is, why? Prior to their death, toxins accumulate in the cells that support the health of photoreceptors: the RPE (retinal pigmented epithelial) cells. This makes sense; but what causes such progressive build-up?

In 2015, thanks to a grant from Alberta Innovates Health Solutions, I hire a post-doctoral fellow from France, Dr. Camille Dejos, whose own mission is to study the interactions between photoreceptors and human RPE cells. In the presence of photoreceptors isolated from Stargardt mice, but not from healthy ones, human RPE cells become sick. Stargardt is caused by mutations in single genes, which code for photoreceptor proteins that cannot fold properly and therefore have an abnormal shape. This shape change means that the diseased protein ends up at the wrong place in photoreceptors and is eaten up by RPE cells, which leads to the accumulation of toxins. Once sick, the RPE cells can no longer support the health of photoreceptors. Here is an analogy: photoreceptors are like someone who has a virus that alone will not harm them, but when passing it to someone else, they then in turn catch a cold. The bad protein alone does not kill photoreceptors; it is its deleterious effect on RPE cells that will lead to their death.

Knowing this, how does one prevent the death of photoreceptors? Many avenues are being explored. Firstly, researchers have tried to replace the diseased photoreceptors using embryonic stem cells. However, in the presence of sick RPE cells the transplanted cells tend to die as well, and the few survivors do not integrate the host retina in a manner that would recover visual responses. My personal experience with stem cells in the retina is that instead of replacing diseased cells, these can deliver survival factors to the remaining host cells. Therefore, they might slow the disease but not reverse it.

A second approach has been to promote the health of photoreceptors such as by feeding them purified fish oil. Some success was observed by Dr. Ian MacDonald in humans afflicted by Stargardt as well as by my lab using mouse models, but larger scale and longer term studies were inconclusive. Nevertheless, Dr. Paul Bernstein from the University of Utah does recommend early implementation of fish oil dietary supplements for Stargardt. One trick to ease its intake is to freeze the soft gels and cut them in half before swallowing.

A third approach entails thwarting the accumulation of toxins. One way to go about it is to limit vitamin A intake. Does it mean eating fewer carrots? Not at all, because carrots only contain molecules (carotenoids) that will be transformed into vitamin A by our body, according to its need. Therefore, if you eat too many carrots, you will turn orange, like a certain American president, instead of accumulating excess vitamin A. However, you should never eat polar bear livers, as they contain pure vitamin A to a point that can actually kill you. I thought I would share this advice, just in case your gastronomic endeavours take you there.

Another way is to prevent vitamin A from being transformed into toxins, such as by using Accutane (yes, the anti-acne cream) or numerous other experimental drugs. Up to fifty percent reduction of toxins has been reported; however, efficacy in preventing vision losses remains under intense scrutiny. A key hurdle is that interfering with vitamin A metabolism has side effects on vision itself. Deficiency in vitamin A, as seen in people with malnutrition, is associated with vision losses. A perhaps less-practical means of thwarting toxin accumulation is to limit light exposure. Consider the social implications of adopting a vampire-like lifestyle!

On a more practical scale, the use of sunglasses is definitely encouraged; you can live as a star who strived to become famous and now ultimately avoids being recognized. Who knows, you might end up signing autographs. It is my opinion that Dagmar does look like a movie star! Finally, a promising avenue opened by Dr. Ulrich Schraermeyer is to promote the removal of the toxin using a drug called Remofuscin. A clinical trial started in 2019 and should conclude in 2021.

The fourth approach bypasses correcting the source of the disease, which is pertinent in late stages once RPE and photoreceptor cells have died. The trick is to genetically transform the remaining cells of the retina so that they can capture light themselves and send signals to the brain. In another blinding disease, at its late stage, Dr. José-Alain Sahel reported recovery of partial vision using this gene therapy method known as optogenetics. The beauty is that regardless of the gene or genes involved, patients can qualify. Therefore, optogenetic therapy could be used in late stage Stargardt. The main objective is time for the brain to learn to process these news signals from the retina. There is accumulating evidence that the brain is quite adaptative; it can learn more than we thought, at any age, as long as it is trained.

The fifth and last avenue is to stimulate cells in the retina electrically, using retinal prostheses. These retinal implants, such as the POLYRETINA developed by Dr. Diego Ghezzi's group, also bypass correcting diseases and are therefore pertinent for late stage retinal degenerations.

In conclusion, many therapeutic avenues exist. How about combining approaches? There is hope in this world. You shall not only see the orange Frisbee as bright as the sun against the green background, as in the play, but will catch it with your own hands and mind.

Wrap-up by William Stell

THANKS TO DAGMAR, we have a vivid description of how Stargardt's disease starts to rob an affected teenager of central vision and how it gets worse and worse as one gets older. The impacts on quality of life and the ability to contribute through work and social activities are formidable, even in someone as resilient and resourceful as Dagmar. Imagine yourself living with Stargardt's in an undeveloped country, and how hopeless it must seem without the resources and supports available in Canada, and without an established and available therapy to arrest the inexorable progression of the disease.

Fortunately, as noted by Dr. Sauvé, research on this and other inherited retinal disorders is very active in Canada and abroad. We may not yet know exactly how to 'fix this', but we can be confident that we will know, before too terribly long. We must realize that even identifying the genetic causes of these disorders, much less developing ways of fixing them, has been with us for only one or two generations — a mere smidgen of human history. New background knowledge, and new ways to prevent vision loss and restore vision, are reported almost daily.

Out of darkness. Fade To Light.

THE LAST DANCE

A Play in One Act

by

Eugene Stickland

INTRODUCTION TO
THE LAST DANCE

—◆—

T HE PROVENANCE of *The Last Dance* is twofold, really. It has to do with a story that I alluded to in the introduction to this volume that presented itself to me in real life (as we are fond to call it), and the opportunity to write a variation of the story and see it produced for a good cause.

To begin with the story, we need to travel back in time to the year 1974 and my hometown of Regina, Saskatchewan. The setting is the gymnasium of one of the older high schools in town, Scott Collegiate. It is the evening of the Senior Prom.

I was at the prom with my childhood sweetheart, Debbie. Deb, as she was known. We had known each other seemingly forever. We went to the same elementary school. In Grade 7 we dated for the first time, all very innocent and naïve. I bought a little ring for her at the old Kresge's store downtown on 11th Avenue. I believe it cost 89 cents. Then we broke up. But then we got back together again. But then we broke up. On and off, on and on. At once point her family moved to a house across the street from our house. We went to the same small high school, in the same grade. It was hard to avoid one another for the most part.

At the prom, she was wearing the wrist corsage I had given her a few hours earlier. We were good enough friends that we didn't need to pretend there was any great romance involved that evening. A couple of times I snuck outside for a drink and to share a joint with my friends. Until finally, I went out and came back in but Deb was nowhere to be found.

It wasn't as grim as it sounds. I knew she'd been seeing one of our classmates. In fact, they eventually

—⦉⦊—

Our conversation [about ALS] could surely be the basis for a play somewhere down the road.

—⦉⦊—

got married and they had a very good life together. And besides, my male friends and I had made plans to engage in some kind of distinctively male rite of passage down by the river (as they say), involving copious amounts of alcohol and other substances and we did that and all ended well.

Fast forward some 40 odd years. I was at home in Calgary one day and I received a friend request from Deb on Facebook. Of course I accepted. She sent me a message and asked if we could talk on the phone. Of course we could. I gave her my number. We hadn't talked since that night at the prom.

She called me. The first thing she said was, "I'm sorry I dumped you the night of the prom." I told her

I had managed to get over it. We had a nice laugh and talked a bit about the good ol' days. The real reason for her call was far more ominous, though. She was dying. She had ALS and had very little time to live. She wanted to say good-bye. That led to a very intense conversation, as you might imagine. I remember thinking at the time that our conversation could surely be the basis for a play, somewhere down the road.

Several years after that conversation with Deb, I met Crystal Phillips at Calgary's literary coffee shop, Caffe Beano. Crystal was at that time heading up the Branch Out Neurological Foundation, an organization dedicated to raising money to support research into the family of diseases that includes MS, Alzheimer, ALS, and Parkinson. Crystal had at one time been an Olympic level speed skater, prevented from competing in the games by the onset of MS. The organization had until that point held athletic events, golf tournaments and cycle tours and the like as their fundraising events. Now they envisioned an art-themed evening called *Your Brain on Art,* proceeds from which would support technology developed by Dr. Bin Hu to assist people with Parkinson. They approached me about creating a play suitable for such an event.

And so I thought back to my last phone conversation with Deb. I imagined a variation of that conversation brought to the stage: a couple of old friends, even sweethearts, coming to grips with the passage of time. The elephant in the room: her having and dealing with the ravages of Parkinson disease.

It was perhaps an act of extreme egoism to present the character representing myself as a world-famous rock star, owner of a small castle in France. As was the case with the architect in *Closer and Closer Apart*, perhaps these plays allow me to live vicariously through the characters I create. Hard to say. But certainly in terms of theatrical appeal, a rock star will always be more interesting than a playwright, hands down.

I am hardly an expert on Parkinson disease, but through the Branch Out Foundation connections I was able to meet with a neuroscientist at the University of Calgary and actually try for myself the technology that Dr. Bin Hu is developing to help people with Parkinson improve their gate. Dr. Hu, with one of his patients, demonstrated the technology at the *Your Brain on Art* event. It is very impressive and helps prevent falls, which is a very serious problem for people with the disease.

I gave very few prompts in the script for the actress, Krista Stephens, who played Leanne. I find in most cases you can't go wrong allowing actors to do their own research and make their own choices. Whatever Krista did in our production was obviously very effective. As she was having a glass of wine after the show, a patron approached her and said, "I think it's great that you still perform, even having Parkinson's." Krista replied, "I don't have Parkinson's. I was acting."

THE LAST DANCE

The Last Dance was commissioned by the Branch Out Foundation to be performed at an event to raise funds for the Ambulosono technology and research. For further information about this technology and treatment, and the work of the Branch Out Foundation, please visit www.branchout.com.

The Last Dance was presented by The Branch Out Foundation's fundraising event on May 17 and 18, 2018 at the cSpace Theatre, Calgary, Alberta with the following cast and crew:

Leanne .... Krista Stephens
Ronny .... Jerod Blake

Direction .... Joe-Norman Shaw
Set and Lighting Design .... Brad Leavitt

The Last Dance

Characters

RONNY: In his fifties. He is a world famous rock musician, along the lines of Bruce Springsteen or Bryan Adams. A big deal. After graduating from HS, he hit the road looking for fame and fortune, and he found both. In this situation, he looks and acts more subdued than he would on stage, especially when he first started out.

LEANNE: Given the fact they grew up together and dated in high school, whatever age RONNY is, LEANNE needs to be the same. She has recently been diagnosed with Parkinson disease. When she moves, she is somewhat slow and deliberate in manner typical of someone with the disease. She may speak a little slowly, initially, and may experience some hand tremors, but a little of this will go a long way so she needn't act out each and every symptom of the disease. She wears a plain dress and slippers — hardly becoming but still we can see the vestiges of a beautiful young woman.

Setting

A room in Leanne and her husband Harvey's comfortable home, simply indicated with a few chairs and a low table.

Situation

They were childhood sweethearts, now in their early fifties. They have not seen each other since the night of the Senior prom. Having reconnected on Facebook, RONNY, who is in town to receive an honourary PhD, has accepted LEANNE's invitation to drop in for a visit.

Lights up. LEANNE is sitting in a chair at the table. She fidgets. She has small tremors in her hands which she quells by holding them tightly together. She fusses with her hair. She gets up and slowly shuffles UPSTAGE and mimes listening at a door. After a moment she obviously hears something and turns and returns to her chair, trying to hurry but really she is as slow as before. She almost falls but finds her chair and arranges herself in it as RONNY enters. They stare at each other a long moment, then he crosses, awkwardly hugs her, and sits in the other chair across the table.

LEANNE: OK, before we say anything, there's something I would like to get off my chest.

RONNY: OK.

LEANNE: It's been on my chest all these years and I need to get it off.

RONNY: OK.

LEANNE: *(Takes a deep breath. She's rehearsed this a million times)* I'm sorry I dumped you at the Senior prom.

RONNY: Oh yeah . . .

LEANNE: You remember?

RONNY: Of course I remember.

LEANNE: So, I'm sorry, OK?

RONNY: OK.

LEANNE: You accept my apology?

RONNY: Yeah. It's OK. I mean, it was like 40 years ago or whatever. So I've managed to work through it. The pain and rejection and all that.

LEANNE:	It was bad behaviour on my part and I'm very very sorry.
RONNY:	We'll find a way to move on and put it behind us.
LEANNE:	Thank you.

Slight pause.

RONNY:	That was actually the second time you dumped me not that I'm keeping track or anything.
LEANNE:	No, it wasn't.
RONNY:	Yes it was.
LEANNE:	No way!
RONNY:	The first time was in Grade 8. You passed me a note in Social Studies. Remember notes? Primitive text messaging. You told me you were in love with Marty and that we couldn't go out anymore.
LEANNE:	Marty?!
RONNY:	Yep.
LEANNE:	I was never in love with Marty!
RONNY:	Well, you claimed you were in the note. Which I still have, by the way. I kept such things in a Black Magic chocolate box. My parents never threw it out. I actually have all my Wolf Cub badges in there as well. I was quite accomplished, as a Cub.
LEANNE:	I find that hard to believe.
RONNY:	It's true!
LEANNE:	Well, whatever. If I said I was in love with him, if I even said that, I may have overstated the matter. We were only 13, after all.

RONNY: I know. I remember I bought you a little ring
           at a five and dime. Remember that?

LEANNE: I do! That was very sweet.

RONNY: And expensive. I think it cost me 79 cents.
           Anyway. It's all good. A lot of water under the
           bridge since those days.

LEANNE: Yes. A lifetime.

RONNY: Literally. A lifetime.

LEANNE: And look at you now. You're famous!

RONNY: That's what they say. But let's not talk about
           that now.

LEANNE: Right.

Slight pause. Suddenly a little awkward.

LEANNE: So Harvey showed you in?

RONNY: Yes he did.

LEANNE: Did you two get caught up?

RONNY: There's not much for me and old Harve to get
           caught up on. We weren't exactly best friends.
           I don't think he likes me too much. I don't
           think he ever did.

LEANNE: He's threatened by you.

RONNY: And rightfully so.

LEANNE: Don't take it personally. He doesn't really like
           anyone.

RONNY: I suppose that's why he became a dentist. So
           he can torture people and get paid for it.

LEANNE: He's a good man. I need him. Now more than
           ever. So be nice.

RONNY: I'm always nice! When was I ever not nice?

LEANNE: Yeah, right.

RONNY: Well, anyway. He let me in.

Slight pause as he looks her over.

RONNY:	So what's going on with you.
LEANNE:	Oh, well. My health hasn't been very good.
RONNY:	I can tell.
LEANNE:	As much as you don't like talking about being famous, I don't really like talking about being sick.
RONNY:	OK . . .
LEANNE:	They say people become their disease, when they get older.
RONNY:	Well, that's understandable, if it's serious.
LEANNE:	I guess . . .
RONNY:	Are you still working?
LEANNE:	No, I had to stop.
RONNY:	You were a vet?
LEANNE:	Yes.
RONNY:	You always loved animals. I remember. You always had a menagerie.
LEANNE:	Yes. But it got to be too much. I had to stop.
RONNY:	Well, I'm sorry this is happening to you.
LEANNE:	It's not fair.
RONNY:	I know.
LEANNE:	Like, why should this happen to me and not to you?
RONNY:	That's an interesting question! I'm not quite sure how to answer that.
LEANNE:	I've lived a good life. A proper life. I was a good vet, I was good with animals. And I raised a family. I cooked good meals, healthy meals. I followed the Canada fucking Food Guide! I supported my husband, put him through university and helped him establish

	his practice. I even started going to god damned church. While you — Ahh, forget it.
RONNY:	No. What about me?
LEANNE:	No, it's petty.
RONNY:	Tell me.
LEANNE:	Well, you spend you life drinking and carousing and doing drugs and hooking up with girls half your age —
RONNY:	Here we go . . . .
LEANNE:	I read *People Magazine*. I know what you've been up to!
RONNY:	Damn! Are you sure that was me they were talking about?
LEANNE:	You should have been dead at 30.
RONNY:	I know.
LEANNE:	40 at the outside.
RONNY:	I know.
LEANNE:	You and that horrible Keith Richards, you'll outlive us all!
RONNY:	He's my role model.
LEANNE:	It wouldn't surprise me if he was.
RONNY:	He is. And he's a friend.
LEANNE:	You've actually met him?
RONNY:	Of course. He sat in on a couple of songs on my last album.
LEANNE:	Jeez, I forget how famous you are. I know you are, intellectually. I know that. But when you're here in my place it's like we're back in high school again and you're just the same goofy guy you always were.
RONNY:	Thanks. I think.
LEANNE:	So, what's he like?

RONNY:	Keith?
LEANNE:	Yeah.
RONNY:	Short.
LEANNE:	Short?
RONNY:	Yes, quite puny, actually.
LEANNE:	One of the great musicians of all time and that's your assessment? Short?
RONNY:	Well, obviously he's great. He's a legend. But when you get to know someone you tend to forget all that. So, yeah. You asked? I told you. He's short.
LEANNE:	OK.
RONNY:	All those Brits are short. Shrimps compared to Canadians and Americans. Something about a shortage of milk after the war. Plus they all have bad teeth.
LEANNE:	And yet we turn them into these giants, when really they are just little men.
RONNY:	Sure, but they're talented. That forgives a lot
LEANNE:	Fair enough.

Slight pause.

RONNY:	You don't really wish me dead, do you?
LEANNE:	No. I have some dark moments. I can't always control my thoughts.
	But I'm glad you're here. I really am. It was nice of you to come over. I can't even imagine how busy you must be.
RONNY:	I'm glad you got a hold of me. We're long overdue.

Slight pause.

LEANNE: How's your mom?
RONNY: Not so well, actually. She's dead
LEANNE: I'm sorry. I hadn't heard.
RONNY: It's OK.
LEANNE: I try to read the obituaries every day. Just to make sure I'm not in there, right? I guess I missed your mom. She was such a nice lady.
RONNY: Thanks. She always liked you. But it was a tough go at the end. Alzheimer's. She didn't know who I was anymore. Hell, she didn't know who she was. She's better off now .... How's your mom?
LEANNE: Dead. Remember she was quite sick even back in high school. She passed away not long after we graduated.
RONNY: I guess I do remember that. How's your dad?
LEANNE: Dead.
RONNY: Oh, Jeez. Sorry.
LEANNE: It's OK. How's yours?
RONNY: Guess!

They laugh, but make themselves stop.

LEANNE: OMG. We probably shouldn't be laughing at this.
RONNY: I know, right?
LEANNE: We're bad.
RONNY: It's the only thing we know for certain: no one gets out of this alive.
LEANNE: True, that.
RONNY: Maybe that explains my behaviour. As long as I can rock, I'm gonna rock. Know what I'm saying?

LEANNE:	Yeah, I do.

Slight pause.

LEANNE:	So, they gave you a PhD??
RONNY:	Yes they did. PhD. Piled high and deep, we used to say.
LEANNE:	Surely not for being an exemplary citizen. Or a good role model.
RONNY:	I hope not!
LEANNE:	So, you're a doctor now.
RONNY:	*(Wolfman voice)* I'm the doctor of love, baby. You're my first house call. You're my first patient. Open up! Let me see your throat!
LEANNE:	Get away!
RONNY:	Ohhhhh, the patient is not cooperating!
LEANNE:	Damn right, I'm not. I have enough doctors in my life without you getting in on the act.
RONNY:	Yeah, but they're not doctors like me.
LEANNE:	Yeah, I know. They're real doctors.
RONNY:	Really? Is it that bad?
LEANNE:	You have no idea. It wears me out just getting to all my appointments.
RONNY:	I couldn't do it. I'd jump off a bridge.
LEANNE:	It's crossed my mind.
RONNY:	How many?
LEANNE:	Doctors?
RONNY:	Yeah.
LEANNE:	Ummmmm, let's see, 10, I guess?
RONNY:	How can there be 10? That's obscene.
LEANNE:	Well, there's my family doctor, obviously. Two of them actually because they work in tandem. Then there's my neurologist who is pretty much my god these days.

RONNY: Serious? A neurologist? Is that like for your nerves.

LEANNE: Kinda. It's a little more complicated than that.

RONNY: OK. So, there's even more?

LEANNE: There's my nurse who basically knows more than everyone else put together. Being sick like this is obviously freaking me out so I'm seeing a psychologist and a psychiatrist, why not? It's free. And then there are all the therapists. And a masseuse. And a chiro. And a naturopath. And a dietitian. Is that 10?

RONNY: I lost count. I don't think I've seen a doctor in ten years.

LEANNE: Really?

RONNY: Yeah. They make me nervous.

LEANNE: Try and keep it that way.

RONNY: I intend to. I've been lucky. I know that.

LEANNE: They all mean well. They're great people, they really are. But it exhausts me accessing them all. It really does. That's become my life, going from one to the other to the other. Harve is so helpful. He drives me everywhere.

RONNY: So, he's good for something, at least.

LEANNE: Be nice.

RONNY: Sorry.

LEANNE: I really miss driving. It gives you such a sense of freedom. You feel so in control. You get all that taken away from you. You feel like you're not in control of anything. Harve takes me out for drives to the country but it's not the same. I want to put the radio on full blast and sing my guts out but you can't do that with someone else in the car.

He gets up and moves behind her, puts his hand on her back, rubs it gently.

RONNY: I didn't know it was so serious. I'm sorry.

LEANNE: Thanks.

RONNY: It's tough, eh?

LEANNE: Yeah. I try to be brave. But it is tough. I can't tell Harve this, but I can tell you: there are days when I dream of checking out, ending it all and it's the most beautiful dream I can imagine.

RONNY: I get that. I feel that too sometimes.

LEANNE: You?

RONNY: Yep.

LEANNE: You've got to be kidding. You have everything anyone ever dreamed of.

RONNY: I guess. But honestly, Leanne, there have been a lot of wretchedly lonely nights. I know. Poor me. No one wants to hear it from me and I can't blame them. But I've lost a lot of friends along the way who couldn't take it anymore. I've lost other friends and lovers. You remember Spider from my first band in high school. He was with me for about five years. Such a happy-go-lucky guy. Then one night he just walked into the ocean with a glass of Scotch in his hand, just walked out like he was in his garden. We all watched him. We thought he was kidding. But he didn't stop, just kept going. We never saw him again. Others take pills, other drugs. There's jumpers and cutters. All manner of methods. It's all very creative, I guess. So it's not just you. Human existence is very difficult. I don't care who you are ...

Pause. He sits down again. She sizes him up.

LEANNE:	So, they actually gave you a PhD?
RONNY:	Yes. For a sustained and significant contribution to the arts and culture of the country. Or words to that effect. Want to see it?
LEANNE:	You have it with you?
RONNY:	Yeah. It was in a big bulky frame. But I didn't feel like lugging that around all night so I just took it out and put it in my pocket.

He takes the degree from his back pocket and unfolds it.

LEANNE:	Wait.
RONNY:	What?
LEANNE:	Wait wait wait wait wait wait wait.
RONNY:	What?!
LEANNE:	You can't just fold up a degree like that
RONNY:	Why not?
LEANNE:	Oh, brother. You've been carrying that around like that since last night?
RONNY:	Yeah.
LEANNE:	Why didn't you just leave it in the frame and leave it in your hotel room?
RONNY:	Right. Oh. Well. Uhmmm, hmmmm. I didn't exactly make it back to my hotel. Room. Last night. You know?
LEANNE:	No, I don't know.
RONNY:	You know ...
LEANNE:	Ohhhhhhhh. Are you telling me you got lucky at your convocation?
RONNY:	Uhhhh, yeah. Yes. That happened.

LEANNE:	Who? How?
RONNY:	Have you ever seen the Registrar at the Uni?
LEANNE:	Not that I'm aware of.
RONNY:	She is sooooo hot.
LEANNE:	Really?
RONNY:	Oh yeah. Smokin'.
LEANNE:	The Registrar at the Uni is smokin' hot?
RONNY:	Yeah.
LEANNE:	So, you're telling me you got lucky with the Registrar? Is that honestly what I'm hearing?
RONNY:	Yep.
LEANNE:	You know, you are . . . I can't even think of the word.
RONNY:	Incorrigible.
LEANNE:	That's the word!
RONNY:	Yeah, well, I'm a rock star. I get that a lot.
LEANNE:	So, what happened? Enquiring minds want to know.
RONNY:	Well, we were having some drinks after the ceremony. You now, the Chancellor and some profs and what not. And I noticed this one chick that kept looking over and so I worked my way around to her and we had a few drinks and it turns out she's a big fan of my last album "Undertow" which was a bit of a flop so I'm always happy to meet someone who actually liked the damned thing.
LEANNE:	She really liked "Undertow?"
RONNY:	Yeah. What's wrong with that?
LEANNE:	Oh, nothing.
RONNY:	I suppose you didn't.
LEANNE:	Not really, no.

RONNY:	You know, it takes as much time and effort to make a flop as it does a hit.
LEANNE:	I'm sure it does, but if you don't mind me saying, I think you missed the boat on that one.
RONNY:	You know what it is?
LEANNE:	No, what is it?
RONNY:	I'm ahead of my time, that's what it is.
LEANNE:	I see.
RONNY:	I'm waiting for the rest of you to catch up.
LEANNE:	If that's what you want to think …
RONNY:	No one sets out to fail. It just happens sometimes. Anyway, she really likes it. She actually has it on vinyl. She asked me if I would sign it for her. So we went back to her place and listened to it and had a few more drinks and one thing kinda led to another... Anyway … *(Pointing to the degree)* Look. They even got my name spelled right.
LEANNE:	I can't believe you folded it.
RONNY:	I like to travel lite. It's no biggee.
LEANNE:	But it's ruined now!
RONNY:	It's just a piece of paper.
LEANNE:	No it's not. It's an honour. It's a great honour. You should take it seriously.
RONNY:	Really, it's not a big deal for me.
LEANNE:	It is for me. And for everyone else.
RONNY:	Well, I'm not everyone else.
LEANNE:	You can be so dense sometimes, you drive me crazy.
RONNY:	What?!

LEANNE: It's not always about you, you know. It doesn't always have to be about you. There are other people drawing breath on the planet, not just you.

RONNY: It's my degree, I can do with it what I want. I could burn it if I felt like it.

LEANNE: You just don't get it, do you?

RONNY: What's to get?

LEANNE: Most of us, almost all of us, 99.9 percent of us, lead pretty ordinary lives. Mundane, by your standards. We get very little recognition, if any. Things like this don't happen to us. They never do. I'm at the point in my life where just walking to the bathroom is a major accomplishment, but there's no one giving me a degree for that. But they do it for you. And rightfully so, you deserve it. And because we all feel that we know you, even people who don't but those of us who actually do, who grew up with you in the old neighbourhood, we share it with you. We share your achievements, your fame even, because we know nothing like that will ever happen to us. We take it seriously, and if you don't, then it invalidates our experience. Maybe even our lives.

RONNY: If it means that much to you, you can have it.

LEANNE: It's not what it means to me that's the issue here. It should mean something to you. It's your home town. You're from here. It should mean something.

She examines it, trying to smooth the creases.

I would try to iron the creases out, but I can't even hold a damned iron anymore.

Slight pause. He watches her. She cries a little, running her hands over the degree. He suddenly feels very small.

RONNY: OK. I get it. Look. When I get back home I'll send them an email and tell them I lost it and ask them to send me a new one. And I'll hang it on my wall.

LEANNE: Really?

RONNY: Yes.

LEANNE: Promise?

RONNY: Yes.

LEANNE: Pinky swear?

RONNY: Pinky swear.

They pinky swear. Slight pause.

LEANNE: So, you actually have a home somewhere

RONNY: Yep.

LEANNE: With walls?

RONNY: Yep. I got walls. And a floor that often enough I end up sleeping on. And a ceiling. The whole nine yards.

LEANNE: Where do you live?

RONNY: You don't want to know.

LEANNE: Try me.

RONNY: I bought a castle. In France. Just a little one.

LEANNE: A modest castle?

RONNY: Yeah.

LEANNE: Does it have a moat?

RONNY:	No, but is has a turret. Two turrets, actually
LEANNE:	What's a castle without a turret or two?
RONNY:	The acoustics are amazing. We recorded our last album there. The one Keith played on . . .
LEANNE:	You know, you've come a long way for a skinny kid from the old north end.
RONNY:	I guess.

Long pause. They look at each other, trying to come to grips with the vast time and space between them.

LEANNE:	So . . . whatever happened to you, the night of the prom?
RONNY:	Ha. Isn't it funny. I can't remember what I had for breakfast but I remember that night so clearly.
LEANNE:	Me too. I did apologize, didn't I?
RONNY:	Yeah, we're good.
LEANNE:	Good.
RONNY:	So I went out for a smoke. Somebody had a mickey of rye so I had a couple of hits of that. Somebody else sparked up a joint. It was a beautiful night, all quite lovely. One of the teachers who was supposed to be chaperoning us got in on the joint.
LEANNE:	Seriously?
RONNY:	Yeah.
LEANNE:	Which teacher?
RONNY:	Oh, hmmmm. What was his name? He taught math.
LEANNE:	Mr. Ball?

RONNY: No, not Mr. Ball. He was a dork. The other one. The cool one. We called him Clark Kent.

LEANNE: Mr. Pickets.

RONNY: Yeah. That's right. Mr. Pickets. He smoked that joint with us.

LEANNE: Nice chaperoning.

RONNY: What was he going to do. It was a tough school, and we were all 17 or 18.

LEANNE: It was a tough school, wasn't it?

RONNY: Yeah. A tough school in a bad neighbourhood. We were poor. We grew up poor. Did that ever occur to you at the time?

LEANNE: At the time, no. It was just what you were used to. It's all you knew.

RONNY: It didn't seem to matter, really.

LEANNE: But if I ever have to eat another fried bologna sandwich ever again, just shoot me will you.

RONNY: Done! Same goes.

LEANNE: So then what happened?

RONNY: When?

LEANNE: That night.

RONNY: Oh right! Well, I got back to the gym, looked around. You were nowhere to be found. One of my informants told me you had taken off with Harvey. I wasn't really surprised. I wasn't even mad or anything, maybe I was relieved. Most of the guys I hung out with had gotten themselves dumped by then. Then there were some like the Beaver who didn't have a date in the first place.

LEANNE: He's one of Harvey's patients now.

RONNY: The Beaver?

LEANNE: His name is actually Lawrence.

RONNY:	I don't think I ever knew that.
LEANNE:	Harvey's got him looking almost normal now.
RONNY:	That poor kid. We rode him hard.
LEANNE:	He turned out OK. He's a judge now.
RONNY:	Really? Well, I hope I never end up in his court room. I'd get the gallows for sure!
LEANNE:	Deservedly so.
RONNY:	Ha ha, kidding right?
LEANNE:	Not really.
RONNY:	Right. Anyway, Deano, Ricky and I and a few others ended up at Turkey's place, down by the river. I know, it sounds like a Bruce Springsteen song, but that's how it was. We more or less drank ourselves into sobriety reminiscing about the good old days — 17 and we felt so old! Waiting for the sun to come up. Which it eventually did. Some of us went for breakfast at Fullers. I remember Deano throwing up in the parking lot.
LEANNE:	He was always so elegant.
RONNY:	No lie. Whatever happened to him?
LEANNE:	No idea.
RONNY:	I went back to my parents' place and wrote "The Dawn of Nothing Special." My first big hit. Changed my life and I wrote it in like half an hour.
LEANNE:	"Stumbling in the same old way Situation normal The shining of the sun's first rays On the dawn of nothing special."
RONNY:	You know it.
LEANNE:	Me and a zillion other people. I wore that album out.

RONNY:	I'm touched.
LEANNE:	It's a beautiful song.
RONNY:	Thank you. I probably thought so at one time too but I've played it so many times over my career I'm sick and tired of it. A week later, me and Spider and the boys drove out to the coast and got some gigs and it just kept goin' and growin'. I only ever came back to see my folks but then I just moved them out to the coast on account of the winters out here . . . So, what about you? What happened to you that night?
LEANNE:	Harvey and I ended up back at his place. Down in his parents' rumpus room. And. You know . . .
RONNY:	No, I don't, actually.
LEANNE:	Yes you do. You know better than anyone
RONNY:	Are you telling me you put out for Harvey?
LEANNE:	I guess I am.
RONNY:	I hope you removed the wrist corsage I gave you first.
LEANNE:	Oh my God. I forgot all about that wrist corsage!
RONNY:	Well, that's quite the outcome.
LEANNE:	You got a problem with it?
RONNY:	Yeah.
LEANNE:	What?
RONNY:	You never put out for me!
LEANNE:	Oh for Pete's sake, that was over 30 years ago
RONNY:	So?
LEANNE:	You got it on with half the girls in North America since then. Not to mention the Registrar!
RONNY:	That's different.

LEANNE: All those heroics and you're bent out of shape about the one girl you didn't get to bang?

RONNY: That's right.

LEANNE: That makes no sense.

RONNY: Yeah, it does, actually.

LEANNE: What sense does it make.

RONNY: I happened to love you.

LEANNE: Oh.

RONNY: Yes.

LEANNE: I see.

RONNY: Yes.

LEANNE: I don't think you ever bothered to mention that, before.

RONNY: I was 17. And scared of it. And too insecure to say anything. But I felt it. Of course I did. I bought you a ring!

LEANNE: You don't know how much it means, to hear that.

RONNY: Really?

LEANNE: Look at me. I'm not exactly an object of adoration these days.

RONNY: You're still beautiful.

LEANNE: Thank you. For what it's worth, Ronny, I loved you too.

RONNY: Really?

LEANNE: I don't think I ever stopped.

RONNY: Then why?

LEANNE: Why what?

RONNY: Why would you dump me for someone like Harvey?

LEANNE: I did what I had to do. You were wild. You scared me. I knew you would never settle down.

RONNY: I might have.

LEANNE: Never.

RONNY: I could have been one of those guys, probably.

LEANNE: What guys?

RONNY: Those guys with the power tools out in the garage. Or in the basement. Whatever. I could have gotten a real job. And a mini van. And a hair cut. And sensible footwear. And all that.

LEANNE: In what dream world do you see that happening? Not this one, that's for sure.

RONNY: Why not?

LEANNE: *(laughing)* Ha! Power tools! You! In your leather pants and your bangles and your chains and long hair, out in the garage making a bird feeder for the back yard! Oh my God. That's the funniest thing ever!

RONNY: I could have been like that, maybe.

LEANNE: Never in a million years.

RONNY: Maybe not . . .

They laugh.

RONNY: I'm probably wearing you out.

LEANNE: I get tired easily, yeah.

RONNY: I know. Harvey told me. He warned me. Sternly. "Don't tire her out, whatever you do."

LEANNE: It's OK. It's so good to see you. RONNY: It's good to see you.

He pulls a flask from his jacket pocket.

Mind if I have a drink?

LEANNE: No, not at all.

RONNY: Want a hit?
LEANNE: Yes. *(taking the flask)* Don't tell Harvey.
RONNY: Our little secret.

She has a drink and hands the flask back.

Here's looking at you, kid.

He drinks and puts the flask away.

Anyway, I guess I have a plane to catch.
LEANNE: What time?
RONNY: Whenever I get there, I guess.
LEANNE: How does that work?
RONNY: Well, it's my plane.
LEANNE: Right. Of course.
RONNY: Keep my degree. It's too bulky to lug around.
LEANNE: You promise you'll get another one.
RONNY: I promise.
LEANNE: Thank you.
RONNY: I'll hang it in a prominent place.
LEANNE: Send me a picture. I want some proof.
RONNY: OK. I will. Now. Before I go . . .
LEANNE: Yes?
RONNY: I feel I am owed something. Something that
           was denied me many years ago.
LEANNE: What?
RONNY: The last dance we would have had at the
           prom. The one we missed.
LEANNE: Dance?
RONNY: Yeah.
LEANNE: Are you crazy? I can't dance. I can barely walk
           without falling over.

RONNY:	You can dance.
LEANNE:	No, I can't.
RONNY:	Yes, you can.
LEANNE:	My legs are made of water.
RONNY:	What are you talking about?
LEANNE:	Ronny, I'm not just a little bit sick. I don't have something that will go away.
RONNY:	OK?
LEANNE:	I have Parkinson's.
RONNY:	Serious?
LEANNE:	Yes.
RONNY:	Why didn't you tell me?
LEANNE:	I don't know. I thought you would come and go and you wouldn't have to know.
RONNY:	You think I don't want to know?
LEANNE:	I don't know. I don't know how to deal with it, OK? I don't know.
RONNY:	You give me shit about my degree, you think people who know and love you don't want to share this with you?
LEANNE:	I don't know.
RONNY:	So it's way worse than you told me.
LEANNE:	Yes.
RONNY:	Tell me how it is.
LEANNE:	You don't want to know.
RONNY:	I do. Go ahead.
LEANNE:	I don't know. It obviously sucks. Some days are better than others, I guess. But it creeps in and takes hold and you just think shoot me I want to die then it relaxes a little but it never really goes away, of course. It's hard to get around, just even to walk anywhere, you're

always worried you're going to fall. There's spasms that just come over you, wrack your body with pain; you wonder what you ever did wrong to have this happen to you. Nights are the worst. I'm afraid to go to sleep for the dreams I could have. The hours crawl by. Can't even read because the print jumps around the page. I won't lie. It's not easy.

RONNY: I'm sorry. That really sucks.

LEANNE: Yes. It does. It really sucks.

Pause. He comes over and hugs her.

RONNY: You have Parkinson's so you think you can't dance.

LEANNE: I know I can't.

RONNY: They have all kinds of research going on, don't they?

LEANNE: I guess they do. It doesn't seem to happen fast enough. But yeah. There's hope things will get better.

RONNY: Well, be that as it may. I've come a long way, and we are going to dance.

LEANNE: I can't.

RONNY: I'll hold you.

LEANNE: What would we even dance to?

RONNY: The last song they played that night at the senior prom. I asked around in the manner of Sherlock Holmes and found out what it was. Kind of an obvious choice, but effective, I thought.

LEANNE: But we don't have any music.

RONNY: That's what you think. I'm in show business, remember? It's the magic of the theatre!

He snaps his fingers over his head and we hear Paul Young's 80s hit, Every Time You Go Away, start to play. He puts out his hand to her in gentlemanly fashion. She accepts it, and gets to her feet. He holds her tenderly and they dance as well as they can.

After the first verse has ended, the lights shift somewhat. He pushes her away. At first she stumbles and shuffles, but as the lights continue to change, she becomes more confident in her movement. She now inhabits the body of her 17 year old self. A light hits a mirror ball. Suddenly we are transported back in time to their senior prom.

They come together again, holding each other. He slides his hand down to her bum and squeezes it. She reaches behind her and slaps his hand away.

Their dance ends up as a full blown balletic pas de deux. As the song ends, they come together in a final embrace as lights fade
to blackout.

We might reasonably think the evening is over, but then from the blackout, a spot hits the mirror ball and we hear the first bars of David Bowie's Heroes. Lights up on LEANNE and RONNY who take their bows. The music continues to build and they dance.

After the first verse, they go into the audience and each brings an audience member onto the dance floor. They all dance together and then select new partners from the audience. This continues until virtually everyone in the audience is up dancing to
Heroes.
And when the song ends, so does the play.

END OF PLAY

—୰—

Author's Note:
Music and the Ending of the Play

Every Time You Go Away *came out in 1985,* Heroes *in 1977. It stands to reason then that if these songs were played at their grad, and they were both 17, they would have been born in the late sixties, and so in 2021 would be in their mid fifties. If the casting is any younger than that, then I would suggest you find appropriate songs for the perceived year of their grad. In the production for* Your Brain on Art, *we weren't able to do the ending as I wrote it. It's a tall order to choreograph a dance on top of everything else when time and funds are limited. I thought it worth keeping in, though, because I believe performed as written, it would be a beautiful spectacle.*

REFLECTIONS ON
THE LAST DANCE

With Crystal Phillips and Bin Hu

—✺—

CRYSTAL PHILLIPS

To THINK THIS ALL STARTED with a coffee conversation at Caffe Beano in Calgary. Eugene Stickland, whenever he lifted his head from writing in his journal with his fountain pen, knew everyone who passed by in the place. We became acquainted, exchanged life stories, and that was the spark that began a new theatre performance and fundraising event — *The Last Dance.*

My personal story starts back when I was a teenager and Olympic hopeful in the sport of speed skating. I was a jock with the following daily routine: Eat—Train—Eat—Nap—Train—Eat—Sleep—Repeat. I *loved* being an athlete and I was on target to make my Olympic dreams come true, until one summer day in 2005...

In a matter of three days, I went from one of the top junior speed skaters in Canada to not walking. I lost feeling from my chest to my toes, lost bladder control and had double vision. A few tests later and I was diagnosed with multiple sclerosis (MS), a degenerative neurological disease with no cure. They said I would probably never speed skate competitively again.

Thankfully, I was stubborn and competitive enough to refuse to accept this prognosis. I quickly dove into the world of both conventional and unconventional healing. I took a painful drug injection every day and was a guinea pig for all forms of therapies to heal my disease-ridden nervous system. Over four years, I climbed my way back to a competitive level in speed skating and qualified for the 2010 Olympic trials. My dream was becoming a reality again until another setback in the pre-Olympic season. I woke up blind in my left eye, a common symptom of MS.

After more tests, I was told my disease was progressing and more aggressive drugs were recommended. The side effects of the drugs sounded worse than the disease itself and I figured that if I was now on track to being in a wheelchair, I had nothing to lose by trying something new.

I decided to go off all of my drugs and treat my disease 'naturally' and more holistically instead of the recommended drugs. Eight months later, I came a few spots off the Canadian Olympic team and twelve years later — is now. I'm in my mid-thirties and thriving with pretty close to optimal health.

This personal experience highlighted gaps in the medical system and filling these gaps became a bigger dream than the Olympics themselves. We needed more scientific validation for some of the less conventional approaches to healing neurological conditions like MS, Alzheimer's, Parkinson's, mental health disorders, epilepsy, and so on. I was inspired to 'branch out' and raise money to fund an entirely new field of study that focused on tech and non-pharmaceutical solutions to neurological disorders. So I retired from speed skating to pursue my new dream of starting the Branch Out Neurological Foundation.

Only problem; my background was skating in circles and not neuroscience or fundraising. I quickly learned the valuable lesson of collecting unlike minds with various strengths to help me. For example, a speed skater meeting with a playwright.

It had been a few years of growing the Branch Out Foundation when Eugene Stickland and I had our coffee conversation. He told me about his close friend who'd developed Parkinson disease and spoke to the suffering his friend endures. This reminded me of a Parkinson's research study that the Branch Out Foundation helped fund. A professor out of the University of Calgary was developing a technology that used music and movement to motivate the brain to change and build new neural pathways. Parkinson patients using this technology were able to walk without the common 'freezing' effect and were now able to confidently leave their house, dramatically increasing their quality of life.

Eugene and I looked at each other with that, *Are you thinking what I'm thinking?* look.

In the following ten minutes we developed an idea to create a play on Parkinson disease. Eugene would write the play, hire and train an actor/actress, and we would feature the play at a fundraising event where we will use various art forms to communicate science and provide inspiration and hope for a healthier future.

A few months later, that ten-minute idea turned into a sold-out event called *Your Brain On Art*. The event raised over $60,000 to accelerate innovative tech and non-pharmaceutical approaches for neurological disorders. It was so loved that we are now planning our Fourth Annual *Your Brain On Art* in Calgary and a fifth in Toronto in 2021.

Thank you to Eugene, the *Your Brain On Art* committees and all the brilliant unlike minds from across Canada who help the Branch Out Foundation move us closer to a world free from neurological disorders.

DR. BIN HU
Suter Professor for Parkinson's Disease Research

Music, Brain and Parkinson's Disease

I AM DELIGHTED to be a contributor to this fascinating book on neuroscience and art. In my academic career as a professor and clinician scientist with a keen interest in music, the brain, and Parkinson's disease (PD), I have had many opportunities to work or interact with writers, journalists, and artists such as Oliver Sacks and Renee Fleming. I first met Mr. Stickland at a fundraising event by Branch Out Neurological Foundation. His play on the life of a Parkinson's patient and her family was truly inspirational and enjoyable to watch. As a talented play writer and lovely companion at the bar, the evening was both memorable and entertaining. At the same fundraising event, I was invited to give a talk about 'Brain, Music, and Parkinson's Disease," which has been a central theme of my research for more than a decade.

There are few forms of arts in human culture that we respond to so tenaciously as music. Music can bring immense feelings of pleasure, the urge of movement, ecstasy, or even a sense of unparalleled altruism and serendipity. Throughout modern history, music has also been documented as a way of relieving human suffering, not the least of which is an eloquent series of books by Oliver Sacks on Parkinsonism.

Parkinson's disease (PD) is a neurological disorder that affects the flow of body movements, thought, and speech, which renders them slow, rigid and jerky.

Bradykinesia, which refers to 'a slowness to initiate walking' and 'gait freezing', is perhaps the most disabling PD symptom. In his book, *Musicophilia*, Dr. Sacks vividly describes how his patient Frances D. responded to music:

> ...music was as powerful as any drug. One minute I would see her compressed, clenched, and blocked, or else jerking, ticcing, and jabbering — like a sort of human time bomb. The next minute, if we played music for her, all of these explosive-obstructive phenomena would disappear, replaced by a blissful ease and flow of movement, as Mrs. D., suddenly freed of her automatisms, would smilingly "conduct" the music, or rise and dance to it.

I believe Dr. Sacks is the very first medical professional who has used his impeccable literal skills to vividly and explicitly portray the miracle effect of music on Bradykinesia. Literature and art can play a pivotal role in disseminating and conveying the discoveries and knowledge to the general public, especially those pertinent to brain and medicine. For artists and playwrights, neurological conditions including autism, Williams Syndrome and Parkinson/Alzheimer diseases, have always been a fascinating subject. For example, many artistic presentations of PD have made their way into movies, for example *Awakenings*, documentaries, and plays like the one written by Eugene Stickland. Nevertheless, based on my personal experience, I consider that the inspiration of scientific curiosity and motivation of artistic pursuits is the most exciting out-come born between the marriage of art and medicine.

I first met Dr. Sacks in Calgary where he was invit-ed to the 2005-2006 Distinguished Writers Program by the Faculty of Arts at the University of Calgary. I vivid-ly remember the night at the River Café where we had a delightful and inspiring discussion on a wide range of topics about the brain, music, and Parkinsonism. Many of the ideas we talked about have subsequently been put into research and clinical tests in a music-based program, Ambulosono. I developed this program after receiving several grants from both federal and provin-cial governments.

Ambulosono walking is a special form of move-ment-music association training. Analogous to piano key playing, in Ambulosono, patients use his or her own step size signals captured by a leg-mounted move-ment sensor to control the playing of highly pleasurable music during outdoor walking. When step amplitudes become shorter than a pre-defined value, music is auto-matically interrupted, thus creating a salient reminder and incentive for the user to actively re-adjust their stride. Hence, during Ambulosono training, music delivery and gait become instrumentally conditioned and behaviorally reinforced, which not only increases patients' awareness of shuffling steps, but it also allows them to become capable of self-correcting Bradykine-sia, thereby regaining the ability of automatic motor control. We found Ambulosono can substantially improve patients' clinical conditions, including gait freezing, walking speed, and, surprisingly, the symp-toms of depression.

Music has now become a central subject in neuroscience research which appears to be a natural shared interest between the art and science communities. As we gain unprecedented understanding on how the brain perceives and processes music and how music can be used clinically to improve speech, memory, and movement, more and more artists are attracted to the opportunities in using the venue of public education to support science and research. A recent example is the Music and Mind program by Mrs. Renee Fleming at The John F. Kennedy Center for the Performing Arts, and a pending exhibition at The National Music Centre in Calgary that features music and the brain. In this regard, *No Harm Done* is very timely and will be a valuable asset as we pursue the synthesis of art and medicine.

PART TWO

DRAMATIST'S

GUIDE

Writing a Play on Commission

For a Special Cause

DRAMATIST'S GUIDE

—⚏—

I HAVE BEEN WRITING PLAYS since 1979, which I now realize means I have written plays in six different decades.
That's a long time to do anything! There have been times
when I could actually make a living writing plays. Other
times, I have had to supplement that income by teaching
others to write plays. I have also written in other forms,
including short stories, poetry, one novel, and six years
writing a weekly column in a newspaper. Some writers have
this kind of versatility, but most prefer to stick to one form.
It's all a matter of personal choice, as well as finding out
where your talent really lies.

My first play came about by rather unusual circumstances. I was offered what seems now a very odd commission to
write a one act play that began as an exercise for a creative
writing class I took at the University of Regina. I think I was
twenty-two at the time. It was a disaster. None of us knew
what we were doing, me in particular. Yet I survived with
a bruised ego and I suppose a desire to try again and see if
I couldn't write something better. Which happened, many,
many times.

Over those years and decades, if I count *The Last Dance*
and *Fade to Light* (which I don't normally because they haven't had full productions, but now that they are published

I feel it's legitimate to count them among the plays of my *oeuvre*), I have written 21 plays. Most of them have been produced more than once, a few of them dozens of times, one of them a hundred times or more. Honestly, I lost count long ago.

When I see these numbers, I have to admit to myself and to the man in the moon that I have been hard-working and diligent all these years, and I am proud of the body of work I have created. Some people have only one play in them. Sometimes it's a really great play, too, but they never manage to write another one. Maybe they don't even want

—⚬—

Of all the arts, I believe
playwriting requires
the longest apprenticeship.

—⚬—

to. If I would look beyond my own genius for a moment, I would realize that more than anything, I was very lucky. I was in the right place at the right time. I had some very talented people who supported my efforts.

With seemingly fewer and fewer production opportunities, theatres closing, pressure to produce only the work of known writers, I worry that few writers in the future will ever get to that number, 21. That's a discouraging thing to have to say to aspiring playwrights, that there's probably no real career in it anymore. (Much the same with journalism, I'm afraid.)

On any account, throughout those six decades when I wrote those twenty-one plays, I taught. Partly this was out of necessity. Writing can be a feast or famine kind of exercise. One needs some stability in one's life. Yet, I would like to think it goes deeper than that. They say that the ability, even the desire, to teach may be engrained in our DNA. My mother was a teacher, as was her mother. Seems like I came by it honestly enough, and I have always thought I do a pretty good job.

The title of this book is, of course, a play on words from a section of the Hippocratic Oath: Do no harm. Doctors have to take this oath, and I sincerely wish teachers had to take it as well. Whenever I start a new class or workshop, my goal is that all the participants will feel as enthusiastic about the subject when the class is completed, hopefully more so, as they did at the beginning. It's never my intention to stomp on anyone's dreams. I feel all I can do is guide my students as best I can to help them write the best piece they possibly can, whether it's a play or a poem or a short story.

My publisher and editor for this book took part in a recent playwriting workshop I taught and thought it would be a good idea to include some kind of writer's guide, along with everything else you find in this volume. It offers me a chance to share my thoughts on how one goes about writing a play, which I have shared with hundreds of writers in workshops over the years, but which I have never written down until now.

I agreed, although reluctantly at first. Of all the arts, and of all the different forms and genres of writing there are, I believe playwriting requires the longest apprenticeship. Playwriting is usually taught over pretty large blocks of time. A university class would likely run for a couple of hours, twice a week for twelve or thirteen weeks. The workshop I currently run for Company of Rogues Actors'

Studio in Calgary goes for about three hours a week for ten weeks. I don't feel I can possibly replicate that process here, but there are a few things I could say that might be of help. So here goes.

1. See plays, read plays

Imagine we are in a workshop together because you want to learn to play the guitar. In my opening remarks, I say that I can't guarantee that you will be playing the guitar like Jimmy Page, but we'll do our best. One of you frowns and puts up your hand.

"Yes?" I ask.

"Ummmm, who's Jimmy Page?" you ask.

"Jimmy Page? Well, he's the guitarist from Led Zeppelin."

Blank stares.

"Led Zeppelin? *Stairway to Heaven? The Rain Song? Whole Lotta Love?* No?"

One of you puts up your hand and explains, "We don't actually listen to music."

Another says, "I sometimes do, but usually piano."

"So, let me get this straight," I say, feeling a massive headache creeping across my brain, "you have never actually heard guitar music, yet you have enrolled in a class to learn to play the guitar?"

It happens more often than you think, especially at the university level where such a class might be perceived as an easy credit, likely with a generous grade at the end of it.

It's a curious phenomenon, but it happens. Given that the theatres around the world have been shut for over fifteen months as I write this, it's likely to become more and more common. It speaks to the allure of the theatre, that people who have never sat in a theatre and watched a play still think they want to learn how to write one.

So, my advice to you is hardly rocket science and it should be thought of as very enjoyable homework. See a play. See a few plays. Try to see a play that's never been done before (we call that a premiere production), maybe written by someone in your own city. Also, see a classic. Shakespeare, or a modern classic like *A Streetcar Named Desire* by Tennessee Williams or *Waiting for Godot* by Samuel Beckett. Don't just watch the movie version. Get up, go out to the theatre. See something live. You will learn more by doing this than from reading anything I have to say about it.

Also, read a play or two. See how the playwright puts the play down on paper. Notice the dialogue, the stage directions, the sound and lighting cues. You can learn a lot by reading plays and you can usually find them inexpensively in secondhand bookstores. If you are reading this because you are from the medical world, one of the best plays I have ever seen which is medically themed is titled *W;t* (as in Wit, but that's how she wrote the title) by Margaret Edson, an elementary school teacher from Georgia. She might just inspire you to write an awesome play of your own!

2. Show us, don't tell us

This is the first holy commandment of playwriting. Of course we go to the theatre looking for actors in the "living moment," as it is known. We look to the playwright to dramatize these moments. We want to see the action unfold before our very eyes in real time. We don't just want to be told about it.

Probably the best example of this can be found (at least in this small volume) in *Closer and Closer Apart*. Melody has tried to express her frustration about her marriage falling apart to her father, Joe.

Her husband's name is Charles, but Joe has always called him Charlie. He comforts her saying "There, there, it'll be OK," and those things we say to people who have come to us for comfort. But as he continues, it soon becomes apparent that in his mind, Charlie is a dog who has run away. It gives the actress playing Melody a real acting moment in her reaction. And of course Joe is oblivious to his own confusion.

This, as opposed to Melody saying, "Gee, father, your brain doesn't seem to be working very well, I think you might have Alzheimers!" That would be telling us. Don't tell us. Put those actors in the living moment and show us that he has Alzheimer.

3. Envision the Space

One of my favourite failed playwriting attempts by a student involved a snowstorm and a parking lot. Two men walk through the snow to get to their car. While one tries to start it, the other brushes the snow off the car. Don't you love the sound of a car that just won't quite start? After "several moments" or so of trying to start the car, the driver gets out and opens the hood. They look at the engine but can't see anything amiss. The driver calls AMA on his cell phone. After being put on hold "for several moments" he gets through and explains his predicament to the unseen person on the other end. He hangs up. They wait in the snow "for several moments." A tow truck arrives. The driver puts on the booster cables and "after several moments" the driver is able to start the car. The tow truck drives away. The car drives away. The driver and passenger talk to each other, but how we are meant to hear them from inside their car will always remain a mystery. Scene.

I actually love it when such scenes are presented because it gives me a lot to talk about, especially when the writer has done absolutely everything wrong, as in this case. The simplest note here is that he's writing a film. (It would have to be a "he.") Sometimes, though, they dig in and want to defend their choices. Fair enough.

So I might have to say, "How do you propose to show a snowstorm on a stage?" He might say something like "You get white stuff and people drop it from above." I see, very clever. I might then ask, "Is the scene that follows this one also set in the parking lot?" "Probably not." "So then what happens to the snow?" "People take care of it." "What people?" "Stage hands and volunteers." "Right."

Further, I might ask, "How do you propose to drive actual vehicles on and off the stage?" "There would be a door." I see. A door to the theatre that a tow truck could fit through. That's some big door! This is going to be done only in the big theatres.

You get the idea.

Even more deadly though than the vehicles and the snow are the "several moments" intervals that pass when nothing whatsoever happens and nothing is said. It's been my experience that audiences like it when something is happening and the characters are saying something, to put it mildly. I have never met anyone who would find it entertaining watching someone try to start a car, let alone pay for the experience.

A variation on this film masquerading as a play motif is another of my favourites. It's a play set in a restaurant. Even better, sometimes an airport! There's the classic film stage direction, "People can be seen passing by with their luggage," or "All around them fellow diners are involved with their meals, engaged in subdued conversation."

At this point (at least by now) I put on my producer's hat. I pretend I am the parsimonious producer and I have to pay for all of this. I might ask, "Who are these other diners?" The answer, "Actors." And so I press, "Actors I should pay for eating a meal and having a subdued conversation?" I move on. "Where is the food coming from? Who makes it? What happens to it at the end of the scene. What happens to all the tables and chairs and all those well-fed actors?" "It all just goes away." "Where?!" "Just away."

You get the idea. None of these are very good choices for a stage play. Let's say my producer's budget is allowing for four actors (of any persuasion), maybe a few chairs and wall hangings and lamps we can scavenge from people's basements. That's about as elaborate as we're going to get. Anything else will have to be created with lights, projections, sound effects, and so on.

But the big shift that needs to happen in the writer's mind is away from film and television to a simpler space, what the British director Peter Brooke refers to as the empty space. In my play *First and Last* we needed to depict an apartment. The play premiered in a space that was more of a lecture hall than a theatre. I asked for an 8 foot x 12 foot carpet to be placed on the floor. This was our apartment. This was our stage. This was our empty space that the action of the play would take place upon.

No one is going to think of driving a tow truck over a Persian carpet — or landing an airplane or anything else. If we have a good honest script with interesting characters, we really don't need much else.

4. Who's Who at the Zoo?

Once we have a reasonable setting in mind, we will want to populate it with characters who are appropriate to that space. There are a few things to keep in mind when constructing a character. First, they are not people. Even if you are constructing a story that happened to you, or to someone you know, or from a historical source, the moment you begin to write them, they exist only as characters that you are creating.

Sometimes we may use a "real life" event as a springboard for our play (as I did in *The Last Dance* in this collection) and yet to adhere to the actual facts may not serve the play you are writing. You need to make some tweaks to reality to create better art. Hence, in that play my autobiographical character is transformed into a rock star who owns a chateau in France, instead of a playwright sitting in a modest apartment in Calgary. Sometimes art is far better than reality!

Then again, some characters are purely intellectual constructs. You see an old woman. She wears a long black coat and walks with a cane. As she walks, she mutters something under her breath. You can't quite make it out. You try to discern something of her demeanor from her eyes but she is wearing sunglasses. She has an aura about her that you find compelling.

Who is she? You don't know, not when she just appears out of the blue like this. Always remember this. Because she doesn't really exist other then in your mind, the only things we can ever know about her have to be what you tell us. And as you can do only so much of that in the list of characters, really we only find out about her from the things she says. Other than that, we know nothing about her.

There is a great adage by the American author Kurt Vonnegut who said, "Every character should want something — even if it's just a glass of water." In rehearsal, good directors will ask actors what their character wants in a scene. Good actors will be able to answer the question. But before any of that can happen, the author needs to ask herself, is it clear what this character wants in this scene? Or in the play? If no one wants anything, there is no urgency or tension to the scene and the play quickly becomes languid, tepid, beige — in a word, boring.

5. He Says, She Says

How we tell the story of course is through dialogue, what the characters say to each other, to themselves, to the audience. You can indicate entrances and exits and notable occurrences on stage (He pulls out a gun, the lights go out, she faints, etc. etc.) Other notes to the actor (her lip trembles, he laughs, she cries, etc. etc.) are not welcome and will not make you any friends with the cast. Seriously, if you are a big fan of stage directions, you should maybe be writing a short story instead of a play. You'll notice that I don't use too many in the plays in this collection.

So, then, dialogue. The things your characters say. One general rule to follow is to ask yourself, with each and every line you write, does this line either reveal something about the character or advance the plot? If not, lose it. The worst thing you can do is have the characters uttering witty things that do nothing but demonstrate that our playwright is a very learned and funny person. (I know, I know, it worked for Oscar Wilde but that was over a hundred years ago and things have changed a little. Besides, he was a genius.)

It's important to keep in mind when writing dialogue

that we don't tend to speak the way we write. Most of us don't speak in complete thoughts. We tend to be disjointed, tangential, fragmentary. If you don't believe me, try an exercise I often assign neophyte students. Sit yourself down in a coffee shop, or any such public place, near a couple of people who are having a conversation. Record it as faithfully as you can. Then go home and type it up. As you type it, try to recreate it in such a way that a couple of actors could replicate it.

Don't worry that it's not about anything — most conversations aren't, really. Don't bother trying to shape it so it has a snappy ending. It's just an exercise. The important thing to take away is a sense of how to write dialogue so it sounds at least vaguely realistic.

We speak, usually, of lines of dialogue. Lines, as opposed to paragraphs. People who speak in paragraphs in conversation are one thing and one thing only: boring. I can guarantee that it's even worse and more boring when it happens in a play. Audiences really don't care for it at all. They will grow restless just before they fall asleep, or worse, leave.

I know it sounds cliché, but think of it as a tennis match. You hit the ball to me. I don't grab hold of it and wax eloquently about the perfections of spheres or the history of tennis or anything else. I hit the ball back. And on and on.

Drama as well as poetry, I think of as vertical writing, prose as horizontal writing. When you are writing prose, you will commonly type until your cursor reaches the right hand margin of your page. The only time it might not would be the final line of a paragraph. Typically prose contains longer, more grammatically complex sentences than either poetry or drama. Leaving poetry aside, dramatic writing rarely makes it to the right margin — at least when it is good and can be said to flow. Our impulse is not to get to the right margin, rather to the bottom of the page.

One final piece of advice about dialogue in this brief primer. Rhythm is meaning. As the stakes get higher, the lines of dialogue become shorter. At the same time, the language becomes simpler, the words shorter. When you have written a good scene where the emotions are high and there is something important at stake, you really don't have to say too much. Give the actors a chance to act.

It's true as well in real life. For many people, the moment in their life when the emotions are strongest and the stakes the highest is their wedding day. (I know this, I've had a few of them.) When it comes to the moment of truth, you are not asked to give a dissertation on the relative merits of monogamy or recite from memory a Shakespearean sonnet. It comes down to two simple and very short words: I do. In some cases: I will.

When it comes to punctuating your dialogue, the only rule you need to remember is to be consistent within your own play. If you really want to emphasize a phrase as I just did above, you might use italics. If the character is meant to scream or shout, then you may wish to do what you do when you're texting: PUT THE TEXT IN CAPITAL LETTERS. As in texting, though, a little of that goes a long way.

Remember always, that unlike a novel, we hear the story only through the dialogue of the characters.

6. Something Should Happen

Action. It's a loaded word with many meanings. It is often misunderstood in the context of writing for theatre or any other form. Most people would probably think of action as in action movies, with lots of car chases and fights and shooting and the like. What fun! But as we know by now, we can't do that on our simple little stage, so we need to tone down our definition of the word as it relates to playwriting.

For our purposes, I am simply thinking of action to mean that something actually happens. (You'd be surprised at the number of student plays I read where nothing, in fact, happens.) Of the plays in this volume, we can see that the action is actually very subtle. *In Closer and Closer Apart,* we can see quite clearly that Melody comes to the realization that her father needs her help. She shows us (as opposed to telling us) that despite the fact that her bags are packed and she's ready to leave, she has to stay, she will stay. She will do the right thing. Despite a new career and good opportunity in a new city, she has to place those plans on hold to look after Joe. Love often calls for sacrifices to be made. To change the course of one's life, to show love and even duty towards a parent — this is what I mean by action.

This of course speaks to another important aspect of character. Assuming you have a central character whom we may refer to as the protagonist, then the hope is that through the events of the play, that character will somehow grow, develop, rise to the occasion, or be crushed by the events that befall him or her — importantly, we see some kind of transformation and the character is different at the end of the play than at the beginning.

I think we can see this in most of the characters in these plays. The one I am particularly proud of in this regard though is Ronny in *The Last Dance.* He comes in as a bit of a spoiled brat, quite frankly, still living out some kind of male teenage fantasy, which is surely our stereotype of rock stars. Yet for him it is a humbling experience to encounter Leanne, reduced as she has been by a debilitating disease. By the end of the play, he seems surely more genuinely human than when he first waltzes in.

7. Plotting Along

The play begins when the status quo is interrupted, and it ends when, as the playwright Arthur Miller said, "all the birds have returned to the wire." Take *Hamlet*, for example. (If you don't know *Hamlet*, which is of course William Shakespeare's masterpiece and in many people's minds the greatest literary work in history, you should. You can find a copy in any used bookstore for pennies, or on the internet for free. And if you don't know *Hamlet*, you can just think of *The Lion King* which follows roughly the same plot line. However, if you are an adult and serious about writing, you may wish to leave cartoons behind and start reading some serious plays, starting with *Hamlet*.)

A lot of people incorrectly think that the status quo is broken in the play when his uncle kills his father and begins sleeping with his mother. Not really. That situation is the status quo when the play begins. What breaks the status quo is Hamlet's father's ghost returning to this mortal coil and telling Hamlet he ought to be doing something about this unfortunate situation, starting with killing his uncle.

The point being that things are as they are, and then something happens to shake up that reality. A couple of the best and most common beginnings to stories of any kind are, "A stranger rode into town," and "Late one evening, there was a knock upon my door."

From this inciting incident, then, a number of things will happen. It is your job as a writer to decide upon what things happen, exactly, and the order in which they happen. If you manage to do this in a skillful manner, the audience will buy into your play. One question that we hope the audience will be asking themselves is "What will happen next?" If what happens next is obvious and predictable, the audience will soon become bored and listless, their minds wondering to who is winning the hockey game or is that wine they like still on sale at Co-op? Build some suspense. Keep them guessing. Be mindful of what information you give out, and when.

Finally, you need to bring this journey to an end. Endings are blessed and accursed things. Blessed when you have one, accursed when you don't. I can't tell you how your play should end. But you should be able to tell me how it ends at a certain point — the earlier in the writing process the better for you and for your play.

All this talk about beginnings and endings — surely you are thinking to yourself, "Wouldn't it be easier to come up with an outline and work from that?" You know, that makes a lot of sense and I wish it worked for me because it sounds like it would be easier. But it has never worked for me so I am reluctant to recommend it.

I think the reason it has never worked for me is that I have discovered, over the years, over the course of writing twenty plays or so, that you find out what your play is about only by writing it. You find out what it is about, what your characters want, what the theme is and your opinion on it, and hopefully where it all will end. Each day of writing will bring you closer to all of these realizations. At least that's how it is for me. I have never been able to predetermine all these things and then write from some kind of master plan outline. It's just not that neat of a process.

8. What's it all about, Alfie?

What is your play about? What big idea are you exploring? What theme are you expounding on that will change the world? I think in some ways the best answer to these questions is an embarrassed or even sheepish, "I dunno."

I have always thought it's not the playwright's responsibility to know what his or her play is about, exactly. Obviously, with the plays in this book, it was pretty clear what they were going to be about, the last two in particular. And yet, in writing the plays and then reading them again years later, I discover they are about more than just their subject areas, and they are about things that I didn't really know about when I set out to write them.

Closer and Closer Apart is obviously about memory, memory loss, Alzheimer disease — these are all givens. Reading it twenty years after I wrote it, it feels to me to be about so much more: roles, responsibility, family, obligation, the nature of love to name a few. I didn't have any of those things in mind when I set out to write it, and yet there they are.

I subtitled *Fade to Light* "A Meditation on Vision." Really though, at heart, it's just a charming little love story. Two characters meet in a park and strike up a conversation. One of the characters happens to be blind. They seem to enjoy each other's company. By the time they run off at the end, hand in hand, it seems reasonable to believe they have fallen in love — ironically what we might call love at first sight. What's that got to do with vision, or vision loss? On the surface of it, not very much. And yet, it seems to work.

Finally, *The Last Dance*. The situation it arose from, my friendship with Debbie and her death, had more to do with ALS than with Parkinson disease. But what is the play about, really? Looking at it now, I would have to say it has something to do with the endurance of friendship and the transient nature of love. I suppose I felt all that, real time, when I spoke with my old girlfriend on the phone all those years later. But I couldn't have articulated it when I set out to write the play. We had loved, we had hurt, but in the end love endured.

So my advice to you, young writer (whatever your age) is not to worry about what the play is "about." Leave it for the critics and academics to figure that out. They are way better at it than you or me. You just worry about what your play is, and trust that the ideas and themes and all the rest if it will be there.

9. The Page

I remember many decades back to the first time I ever tried to write a play. I know some of you will find this hard to believe, but I wrote my first ever play on a typewriter. Not because I was being all cool and retro — that was the technology then. I think it was 1978. I don't think computers became commonplace until the mid-eighties.

In the days before the personal computer, there was no easy way to find a template for what a play script might even look like. I managed to find a book on different formats and styles for various forms of writing, including playwriting. I followed the format I found in there at first, and then over the years, first on the typewriter and now on the computer, I created a style of my own which you can use or modify as you see fit.

In my mind, the most important thing to keep in mind with the design of your script is readability. If your play is ever produced — and that is the goal of the exercise, after all — that means that actors are going to be lugging your script around the rehearsal hall as they learn their lines and the blocking from the director. If the font is too small or the lines too close together, it is difficult to find out where you are on the page as you move around, trying new things.

To this same purpose, actors will often write movement notes, crosses, other actions suggested by the director on the page, so there should be plenty of white space on the page for them to do so. If your writing is tight and for the most part vertical this should not be a problem.

The first thing I do is type my title on a page by itself and then find the font that seems to match the vibe of the play. The font I am happy with these days and that I am using to type these words is called Bell MT. (I have no idea what font my publisher will use for this book; it will almost certainly be something other than that. (*Publisher's note: the book is set in Minion Pro.*) Garamond is another personal favourite. By no means should use a sans serif font like Calibri which for reasons unknown to me is the default font on Word.

Once you have decided upon a font, you will want to default to 12 point text and set the line spacing to 1.5.

I employ a three-margin system. The left margin is for the name of the character speaking, the second is for dialogue and the third for stage directions. I also put the stage directions into italics. I hold these margins for as long as the dialogue or stage directions lasts so it never comes all the way back to the left margin.

At this writing, I don't know how the plays will be designed in this book. What I am suggesting here is good for a manuscript format.

Here's a brief sample:

> *Eugene enters the room SR, throws his coat across the end of the couch, sits down, looking at his phone. Carol is sitting in an armchair SL reading a very large book.*

CAROL: Hello, darling.

EUGENE: Hello, love.

CAROL: How was your day?

EUGENE: Long, tiring.

CAROL: Poor baby. Let me get you a nice martini. Surely the poor baby deserves a great big martini after such a difficult day!

> *She crosses to the sideboard, pours a martini from a stainless steel shaker, brings it to him.*

EUGENE: Thank you.

CAROL: *(Hesitates a bit, then, matter of factly)* Eugene, It's no use. I can't go on like this. I want a divorce.

EUGENE: Ok . . .

To be continued. If you are curious, there is no Carol. There is no sideboard. There have been a few divorces and more than a few martinis, but I was just doing what writers do and making it up. It's not so hard. Try it yourself, you might just like it!

10. Writing on Demand

Somewhere across town, in a well-appointed living room of a fine house, or the board room of a not-for-profit organization, a committee is being formed, an event organized, a gala evening envisioned, the generation of much-needed funds anticipated. What will it be? A golf tournament? A fashion show? And then someone says, "Why don't we commission a play and have a gala evening in the theatre?!"

The next thing you know your name is on a white board or a flip chart along with several others. Then it is remembered that one of the names swears way too much and another is a terrible writer and another drinks and another actually died years ago and soon only one name remains and it is your own name and soon enough they come looking for you.

The good news is they want to pay you. Believe me, I've done this kind of thing in other circumstances only for the money, but it is ideal when the cause for the benefit is a good one, as was the case with the plays that found their way inside this book.

You are always happily surprised that the payment settled upon is actually quite generous. You wouldn't want to charge very much if your fee was coming from the money being raised for research, the evening's take, as it were. You're reassured that there are various pools of money lying around for such things, and that your fee would be taken from one of these pre-existing pools and so would not diminish the total for the evening.

Thus assured, the writer warily listens to what the producers have in mind. I would suggest that if an idea doesn't pop immediately into mind that you decline the enterprise entirely. If nothing springs forth instinctively, I'm not sure how much deep or even strenuous thinking will help change the situation. So with a vague idea and some money in your pockets, you set out to write something that will contribute to "an evening no one will ever forget."

After avoiding the issue for as long as you possibly can, soon enough the deadline looms. Your instinctive idea seems increasingly feeble. You know nothing about this subject, far less than the average person on the street. Far less even than some intelligent dogs. Of course, everyone in the audience will know far more about the subject than you ever will. What were you thinking saying yes to this? You stop sleeping. You lie awake feverishly tossing and turning. You start attending church again.

You get the idea. It is a very tricky assignment. One wants to know something about the matter at hand, but maybe not too much. It seems to me that if you know too much, your characters will become little more than case studies and lose something of their humanity. Remember, we are more than just the sum total of our symptoms. We may have a disease but we are not the disease. So in this regard, a little research goes a long way.

Another thing to be aware of is your potential audience. Fundraisers have their own kind of audience, quite unlike any others I have seen. First of all, they have paid all kinds of money to be there. They have the right to expect to be engaged and even entertained. There is generally no shortage of wine flowing around pre-show, so you can also assume they will be a little (or a lot) liquored up by the time the proverbial curtain goes up. As a result, no matter how serious the reason for them being there (ie, a debilitating disease) they are going to want to laugh. I'm being quite serious when I say you better have some humour in your short play or you'll lose your audience and you will have contributed to "an evening no one will ever remember."

Obviously, you will have to contact someone to produce the play. You can think of the event organizers as the executive producers — they will write the cheques, drawing funds from their various pools. But you will need to find a producer/director. This person will cast the play, find the designers, take care of all the technical aspects of production, rehearse the play and have it all ready for the big night. It's a lot to ask someone for probably not a lot of money, and for a one-off performance at that.

—∞—

Let there be one good laugher
in the audience
who gets my jokes.

—∞—

As the lights go down on the big night, you will likely find yourself standing somewhere at the back of the theatre. I suggest you bow your head and say a little prayer to the theatre gods that might go something like this:

Dear gods, please, please, please let this work. Let the actors remember their lines. Let there be no technical foul ups. Let there be one good laugher in the audience who gets my jokes. Just this one time, dear gods, and I swear I will lead a better life in your service from this day forward. Amen.

11. Final Thoughts

These rather tangential notes (some might say "ram-blings") are meant to be a guide, or maybe even an en-ticement or invitation, for you to write a play of your own with at least a tiny notion of how you might rea-sonably go about it.

If I have piqued your interest, I advise you to find a playwriting workshop or circle or class in your area. These are always being offered through various sup-port groups and colleges and writers groups. Most provinces and states have playwright support orga-nizations that can answer all of your questions. (In Alberta, the organization is called the Alberta Play-wrights Network. They would love to hear from you.)

Writing plays is a lot of hard work. It's a lengthy process. It's not uncommon to write ten or even more drafts before you think it is finally right. Once you have written it, there is no guarantee it will ever be performed. The truly vexing thing I find with it is that the knowledge one gains from writing a play isn't nec-essarily accumulative. It seems every time out (for me, at least) is like the first time. I have no clue of how to proceed. I feel I have nothing to say and no skills to say it with. It can be very bleak terrain indeed.

But if you trust the adage that we find out what the play is by writing it, if you can find the courage to set pen to paper, or to open a file on your comput-er, and write something, anything, you might just find that it starts to make sense. It doesn't matter if what you write is the beginning of the play. It might end up somewhere in the middle. Eventually you might throw it away and not use it at all. The main thing is don't just think about it — start putting words on the page.

If you can do this three or four times, you might just discover something taking shape in the murky mists of uncertainty. And you may find yourself eventually at the point where you can't wait to get back at it again and move it a little further along. In this manner, eventually, it might even take years, you may just find that you have written a play. And with a bit of luck and good fortune and some machinations of the theatre gods, you might actually see your play produced on stage.

I hope that will happen for you some day, in a theatre big or small — it hardly matters the size. Applause is applause, after all. If anything I have written here helps you along the way, then I will have considered it time well spent.

Good writing!

ACKNOWLEGEMENTS

—⚊—

The author wishes to thank all of the original
cast and crew members for all of these plays,
and in no particular order special thanks to
Dagmar Jamieson, Crystal Phillips,
Meagan McKenzie, Johanne Deleeuw,
Bob White, Joe-Norman Shaw,
Aaron Coates, Will Lawrence
and, as always, my beautiful daughter,
Hanna Stickland.
Also, thanks and kudos to Lorene Shyba for
having the vision to bring this book into the
world and for her tireless work and ongoing
belief in Canadian and Indigenous authors.

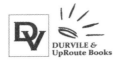

**DURVILE &
UpRoute Books**

Books in the Every River Literary Series

Series Editor: Lorene Shyba

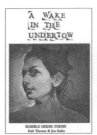

A Wake in the Undertow: Rumble House Poems
Rich Théroux & Jessica Szabo

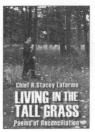

Living in the Tall Grass: Poems of Reconciliation
Chief R. Stacey Laforme

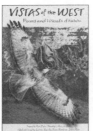

Vistas of the West: Poems and Visuals of Nature
Foreword: Doris Daley
Editors/Curators:
Lawrence Kapustka, Susan Kristoferson, Lorene Shyba

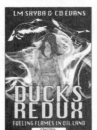

Ducks Redux: Fueling Flames in Oil Land
LM Shyba and CD Evans

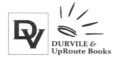 **DURVILE &
UpRoute Books** Durvile.com

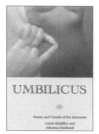

Umbilicus: Poetry and Visuals of the Sensuous
Carrie Schiffler & Johanna Stickland

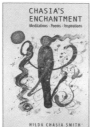

Chasia' Enchantment: Meditations, Poems, Inspirations
Hilda Chasia Smith

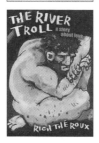

The River Troll: A Story About Love
Rich Théroux

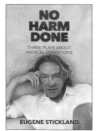

No Harm Done: Three Plays About Medical Conditions
Eugene Stickland

ABOUT
EUGENE STICKLAND

—▨—

BORN IN REGINA, SASKATCHEWAN, Eugene completed an MFA in Theatre at York University, specifically in playwriting and dramaturgy. He moved to Calgary in 1994 at the time of his first major production at Alberta Theatre Projects of the hit play *Some Assembly Required,* which went on to have over a hundred productions worldwide. He wrote nine more plays following that during a ten-year residency at ATP. Following his time at ATP, Eugene wrote a popular weekly column for *The Calgary Herald* and in 2015 he published his first novel, *The Piano Teacher,* which received the W.O. Mitchell Award. He lives alone in the Beltline neighborhood in Calgary, Alberta.